Fitness One Day at a Time

Fitness One Day at a Time

Overcome the nine most common barriers to exercise

Tim Lencki

iUniverse, Inc.
New York Lincoln Shanghai

Fitness One Day at a Time
Overcome the nine most common barriers to exercise

iUniverse, Inc.

For information address:
iUniverse, Inc.
2021 Pine Lake Road, Suite 100
Lincoln, NE 68512
www.iuniverse.com

ISBN: 0-595-32260-3

Printed in the United States of America

Acknowledgements

Above all, I would like to thank my Lord and Savior Jesus Christ for giving me the experience, knowledge and desire to write this book. All that I have and all that I am I owe to Him. His purpose for my life is the driving force behind all that I do. I will continue to give Him glory and praise until the day we meet in heaven.

To my mom and dad, who've been by my side and supported me in everything I've done, I thank you. You are a constant source of encouragement that has made me who I am today. I can only hope to provide that same love and encouragement to my son Noah as he grows up.

To my wife Jill, I thank you for tolerating the long hours and late nights I put forth to complete this book. Your effort to provide a quiet house for me to work in didn't go unnoticed.

To Nancy, my editor and proofreader, thank you for the hours you spent making sure my punctuation, grammar and sentence structure are acceptable to publish.

Disclaimer

Starting an exercise program creates a new stress in the body. Everybody responds to this stress in a different way. I suggest you consult with your physician prior to beginning an exercise program or implementing the suggestions made in this book. This is especially important if you have a history of heart disease, diabetes, a joint condition, or are overweight.

Contents

Preface

Making a Difference in Your Life

My desire to write this book came as a result of many years of hearing people make excuses why they can't start an exercise program.

As of 2004 I've spent 14 years in the fitness industry, with many of those years selling health club memberships. During that period I've heard just about every excuse imaginable.

Not only have I heard excuses why a person can't start exercising, but also the excuses why they quit exercising.

I get so frustrated. I'll spend time talking with a person about why they are thinking about starting an exercise program in the first place. They'll go into a lengthy explanation of how they are out of shape, have a family history of heart disease, or desperately need to tone up. After all this, they decide they have to think about it! What is there to think about? They just explained to me why they need to exercise and how important it is for them to see results, yet they have to think about it. I just want to grab and shake them, saying, "Listen to yourself! You just told me how badly you need to exercise and that you need to get started; what are you waiting for?" Being the professional that I am, however, I restrain myself and politely allow them to give it some thought.

It is for this reason I chose to write this book. I've chosen nine of the most common excuses I've heard over the years and developed some ways to overcome them. By no means are these the only reasons why people don't exercise; however, I feel these are the ones that get used most often.

As an exercise physiologist and certified personal trainer, I know how important exercise is. Daily I read how disease and illness in our society can be reduced with just a little time spent exercising. To see people walk away from exercise when I know they truly need it is difficult.

I want to make a difference in people's lives. I want people to know how incredible exercise can make them feel. How it helps provide a higher quality of life, one that can be enjoyed for years to come.

So in this book I will show you how to overcome the obstacles that keep you from experiencing all that exercise can do. All I ask from you is to have an open mind and a positive attitude. When you come across a barrier that you have been struggling with, take extra time to read about it. Think about how it is relevant to your situation. Once you've read it, immediately apply the solution I offer here.

I'm excited that you made the choice to purchase this book. This could be the start of something that will not only last a lifetime, but a lifetime that lasts.

CHAPTER 1

Should I Be Reading This Book?

"If you can find a path with no obstacles, it probably doesn't lead anywhere."

~ *Anonymous*

If you are a living, breathing human being you've undoubtedly had to overcome some adversity in your life. Am I right? What type of adversity was it? Maybe you lost your job or were in an accident where you had a lengthy rehabilitation process filled with setbacks. For some, moving up the corporate ladder presented obstacles that were difficult to overcome. Still others are trying to escape financial difficulties. Whatever situations you face, I'm sure they can be overwhelming at times.

Rest assured your labor is not in vain. Look at it as Booker T. Washington did when he said, "Success is not measured by the position one has reached in life, rather by the obstacles overcome while trying to succeed."

When it comes to starting and sticking with exercise, the obstacles can be many. As an exercise physiologist and personal trainer, I've worked in the fitness industry for over 14 years. I've learned, heard, and read about almost every obstacle known to man when it comes to exercise. It's these barriers that keep people from being physically active. Understanding which barriers you face and learning strategies to overcome them are the keys to making exercise a part of your life. And that's what it is all about...making exercise a part of your life.

This is not an easy task. The Centers for Disease Control and Prevention released a report in May 2003 showing that only one in five American adults engage in a high level of physical activity, and 25% of American adults engage in little or no regular physical activity.

Where Do You Fit In?

Harvey Lauer, president of American Sports Data, Inc., in a study conducted for the International Health, Racquet & Sportsclub Association: *A Comprehensive Study of American Attitudes Toward Health Clubs and Physical Fitness*, identifies four levels of fitness conscious-ness. The study sought to identify people's physical activity levels along with the importance they put on exercise. As you read through these descriptions, think about where you place yourself.

> **Fitness Fact**
> _____
>
> **Only 1 in 5 American adults engage in a high level of physical activity.**

People in the first level are called the "nonbelievers". They don't think exercise is important. They make up only 2% of the population.

Those in the second level are called the "indifferent." They make up about 16% of the population and feel that exercise is important, but just don't feel the need to get involved.

The third level comprises the largest population, totaling 63%. They are called the "uninitiated believers." They know exercise is important, but are inconsistent with physical activ-ity. To their credit, however, they say they would like to partici-pate more than they do.

Finally, we come to the population called the hard-core par-ticipants, otherwise known as "gym-rats." Hard-core partici-pants make up 17% of the population. These are people who consider exercise very important and participate on a regular basis. They have made fitness a part of their lives. No matter what they do or where they live, exercise will be essential to them. They have learned to overcome the barriers we will be dis-cussing in this book.

Were you able to place yourself in one of these categories? If so, which one?

If you placed yourself in the category of nonbeliever, indiffer-ent or uninitiated believer, then you are reading the right book. You belong to the more than 80% of the American population who need to make fitness a consistent part of their lives. You are in the majority! Wow, cool, huh? Not quite! This is a majority you don't want to be in.

The Unhealthy Majority

Being among the 80% of people who don't make exercise a regular part of their lives is flirting with disaster. The health statistics are staggering.

An inactive lifestyle and poor diet contribute to nearly 300,000 deaths each year in the United States. The sad fact is that 40% of all deaths result from behavior patterns that are lifestyle-related. That means you have a choice!

As of 2003, the government reports that nearly two-thirds of Americans, or 130 million adults, are overweight, with nearly one-third, or 61 million, considered obese. Obesity is defined as an excessively high amount of body fat or adipose tissue in relation to lean body mass. The Centers for Disease Control and Prevention predict that by 2010 obese people will make up 40% of the population.

Living a sedentary lifestyle, one where exercise is not a part of your regular routine, leads to becoming overweight. People who are overweight have a higher risk for getting

> **Not exercising is like smoking a pack of cigarettes a day!**

coronary heart disease, type 2 diabetes, high blood pressure, osteoarthritis, respiratory problems and some types of cancer. The health risk posed by physical inactivity is almost as high as cigarette smoking. I once heard that if you don't exercise, it's like smoking a pack of cigarettes each day! I believe it, too!

Cardiovascular disease is the number one killer of men and women in the United States today. It takes the lives of over one million people each year. Every 33 seconds someone dies from heart disease.

Cancer is the second leading cause of death in the United States, taking the lives of nearly a half million people each year. One in four deaths result from cancer.

Seventeen million people currently have diabetes, with another 16 million in a pre-diabetes state. Each year there are a million new cases of diabetes reported.

All said and done, in 2002, Americans spent an estimated $92.6 billion on medical problems associated with being over-weight or obese.

There Is Hope

My intent with these statistics is not to preach, lecture or nag so as to shame you into exercising. Rather, it's to make you aware of what is really happening in this country today.

It's clearly evident that Americans need to become more physically active. I recently read an article titled "Countdown to Get Active America!" in a monthly journal called *Club Business International*, which is put out by the International Health, Racquet & Sportsclub Association (IHRSA). It talked about a program IHRSA started to help people in this country get more active. The article started with an eye-opening statement worthy of repeating. It said, "Each day, the need becomes more obvi-ous. The nation seems caught in the deadly grip of increasingly sedentary and self-indulgent lifestyles, which are taking a terri-ble toll on the public's health and threatening its very longevity."

Our country is truly facing a dilemma. The good news is that you can choose the lifestyle in which to live. You've already made a great choice by purchasing this book. You've made the effort toward getting started with an exercise program. I applaud you for taking the first step.

Regardless of your age or past experience with exercise, it's never too late to start. I want to tell you a story about an indi-vidual I admire greatly. He happens to be a client of mine. His name is Dick.

Dick led a very active lifestyle, participating in many physical activities over the years, his most treasured activity being golf. Dick belonged to numerous golf organizations, played a big role in the organization and operation of his local country club, and won a few local golf titles. If Dick wasn't out with his foursome on men's day, he was hitting golf balls on the driving range to improve his game.

It wasn't until later in life that I met him. I was able to con-nect with him through his son, who was also a personal training client of mine. They decided it would be a good idea to incorporate another type of physical activity into Dick's life, as golfing was becoming more difficult due to age. So, at 86, Dick began strength training for the first time.

What I've admired over the years of training Dick is his desire to exercise. If I have a conflict that requires me to cancel his session, he is quick to find an alternate time. In all the years I've been his trainer, I could count on one hand the number of sessions we've missed.

Remember, Dick was 86 years old when he started! Most people at that age, if still alive, aren't thinking about what strength training exercises they'll do next, but whether or not they will have the strength to get out of bed.

Dick's attitude toward exercise is encouraging and inspiring to anyone contemplating an exercise program, regardless of age. Sure, he's had some setbacks over the years, but none have stopped him from continuing what he started.

Now, as Dick approaches his 90th birthday, he continues to strength train with me three times a week. He is an inspiration to me and has proven that you are never too old to start exercising. Making the choice to incorporate a new type of physical activity in his life has allowed him to spend a little more time on this earth with those he loves.

I'll Do My Part

Now it's my turn to help you out. This book is designed to give you the tools you need to make exercise a part of your life. Read it in its entirety, even if you have trouble with only certain obstacles. The journey to making exercise a part of your life is long and may be filled with adversity. However, you can overcome it. You will overcome it! Once you do, you'll wonder what on earth took you so long to get started.

CHAPTER 2

Why Do People Fail at Exercise?

*"Success isn't built on success. It is built on failure
and frustration, sometimes catastrophe, and learning
to turn it around."*

~ Sumner Redstone

Failure is a subject not many people care to talk about. After all, who wants to be associated with failure? To fail means you blew it. You lost. You screwed up. Or does it?

In 1955 Johnny Unitas was drafted number nine from the University of Louisville by the Pittsburgh Steelers. That same year he was cut and played semipro sandlot football for only $6 a game. If you're familiar with the NFL, you know that Johnny Unitas didn't give up. The following year he went on to play with the Baltimore Colts, eventually leading them to championship seasons in 1958 and 1959. He also played in 10 pro bowls and was MVP in three of them.

If it weren't for Walt Disney's enthusiasm and willingness to persevere we wouldn't have ever heard of Mickey Mouse and Disneyworld. His initial experimentation with the animated film, *The Alice Commodities,* was a complete flop. When he was 22, his company went bankrupt. Walt Disney never gave up and is now considered an American icon.

How many of you Elvis Presley fans knew he was fired from the Grand Ole Opry after one performance in 1954? Elvis kept singing and the rest is history.

For those of you who like to "fly the friendly skies," be thankful that Orville and Wilbur Wright didn't give up and stick with only the bicycle business. In 1903, four years after they experimented with their first flying machine, history was made in

Kitty Hawk. It was thanks to their obsession and belief in themselves we now can get from one end of the country to the other in a matter of hours.

Thomas Edison patented 1,093 inventions in his lifetime. How many failures do you think he overcame in the process? If Edison had given up one failure short of his greatest invention, we would all be in the dark.

These and many other greats are true examples of why you can't let failure haunt you. Louis E. Boone says it nicely: "Don't fear failure so much that you refuse to try new things. The saddest summary of life contains three descriptions: could have, might have, and should have."

> **"Many of life's failures are experienced by people who did not realize how close they were to success when they gave up."**
> **~ Thomas Edison**

If you've failed at exercise before or have failed to start, become a walking testimony and do what many who have gone before you did...don't give up.

Why People Fail at Exercise

In the first chapter we looked at some of the statistics regarding exercise dropout rates. It baffles me how something that should be so important in our lives has such a high failure rate.

Over the years I've worked in the health club industry I have seen failure happen time and time again. People have such great intentions to start exercising only to see it all dissipate in a matter of weeks. What is it that causes people to fail? What are the barriers that so many people can't seem to overcome?

That is the question I intend to answer in this book. I've identified some of the most common barriers to starting and sticking with an exercise program. In this chapter I'd like to preview some of those barriers and get you thinking about which ones are giving you the most trouble. Then we will focus on each one in detail for the remainder of this book. Let's take a look and help you prepare to overcome!

1. *A Negative attitude will get you nowhere*

It is amazing how powerful attitude is in our life. Charles Swindol once said, "The longer I live, the more I realize the impact of attitude on life." He goes on to say, "The remarkable thing is we have a choice every day regarding the attitude we will embrace from that day...we are in charge of our attitudes."

If you have a negative attitude toward exercise it's because of a choice you've made. You can't blame it on circumstances, limitations or other reasons. If it is to be it's up to me. Your attitude will determine your actions and these actions will determine your accomplishments.

If you try to start an exercise program with an attitude that says you're doing it only because you should, it will lead to failure. Famous motivational speaker Zig Ziglar says, "Feelings follow actions. So when you don't really want to or feel like doing

> **"A human being can alter his life by changing his attitude."**
> **~William James**

what needs to be done—do it and then you will feel like doing it." What Zig is saying is that sometimes you just have to start doing something in order to change the way you feel about it.

Once you get started with exercise and begin to see the positive effects it provides your attitude will quickly change. When it does you'll be amazed with the progress you make.

2. *Exercise and I aren't a good fit*

A lot of people are very self-conscious when it comes to exercise. Being overweight plays a major role in these feelings. These people simply don't feel comfortable in a setting where exercise takes place. It's the fear of being in front of others that is intimidating. Are you one of them? When this is the case, you are faced with a barrier such as "where am I going to work out?"

People are also intimidated by exercise because they don't know what to do. In a study conducted by Peg Jordan, spokeswoman for the Aerobics and Fitness Association of America, 1,880 people were interviewed regarding their motivation to exercise. She discovered that more than 80% saw exercise as "too scientific and too complicated...so that beginners risked exposing their incompentency and ineptitude." These fears are real and can result in the abandonment of exercise.

In Chapter 3, "I Don't Know Where to Exercise," I'll discuss options you have regarding where to work out and examine what options are best for you. We'll also look into the qualities of a great personal trainer and how one can be of assistance to you.

Chapter 4, "I Don't Know How to Exercise," will outline what you need to know about designing an exercise program. It will cover the three important components of exercise: cardiovascular, strength, and flexibility training.

3. A weak commitment just won't cut it

Without commitment don't expect to accomplish anything of great value. Johann Wolfgang von Goethe, one of the most recognized writers of modern time, put it this way, "Until one is committed, there is hesitance, ineffectiveness and the chance to draw back...not committing will kill countless ideas and splendid plans."

If you want to succeed in making exercise work in your life you must be committed to it. You have to give it more than just a few weeks to work. Change doesn't occur as quickly as you may like. Committing to exercise 100% by making it a habit will help you overcome barriers to exercise success.

> **Commitment is the key to long-term success.**

To help you commit to exercise read Chapter 5, "I'm too Inconsistent With Exercise." We'll look at ways you can make exercise a habit in your life.

Chapter 10, "I Can't Afford to Exercise," will discuss some typical spending habits, costs involved with beginning an exercise program and, finally, look at how small changes in the way we spend money can provide the extra money to start an exercise program.

4. No goals, go glory!

Setting goals provides you with a sense of purpose. They help give you the desire to "get going." Basil S. Walsh made it simple when he said, "If you don't know where you're going, how do you expect to get there?"

Having specific goals will give you direction. Without them, how do you know where to go? It's like traveling to an unknown place in your car without a road map. Goals help determine your priorities that will keep you on track toward succeeding. And the success I'm speaking of is being able to make exercise a part of your life. Once you do this, all the little things like losing weight, toning up, and increasing strength and size come more easily.

What is one of the most powerful motivators you know? For many people it is achieving success. Setting a number of small goals and achieving them on a regular basis is very motivating and can keep you focused on the larger goal at hand. When it comes to exercise, doing this is not an option but a requirement. I can guarantee you will face setbacks, lack of results, and times when working out is last thing on your mind. Good goals help you overcome these setbacks.

> "Obstacles are those frightful things you see when you take your eyes off the goal."
> ~ Hannah More

In Chapter 7, "I'm Not Motivated to Exercise," I'll show you some steps to take that will help you get motivated to exercise. We'll look at the importance of casting a vision along with five steps necessary to set goals that enable you to see your vision become a reality.

5. Focus or fail!

Let's face it, there are times when exercise can get a little boring, right? In order to really focus on something, you need to be passionate about it. Passion is defined as powerful emotion or boundless enthusiasm. Whoa! Does anybody have boundless enthusiasm for exercise?

You're probably thinking, "How can I get passionate about something I find boring?" In Chapter 9, "I Find Exercise Boring," we'll look at some ideas you can use to make exercise a little more enjoyable. You may be surprised at what I have to say. You'll also get a chance to read testimonials from people who find exercise enjoyable. It is my hope that, through the testimonials and my ideas, you'll see exercise in a different light, making it easier to stay focused and possibly develop a passion for it.

Before anything can happen, however, you need to take action. Action can lead to passion. Herman Cain, author and CEO of Godfathers Pizza, Inc., agrees: "Success doesn't lead to happiness. Happiness leads to success. If you love or have passion for what you are doing, you will be successful."

6. Taking shortcuts will lead to failure

Fad diets and promises of exercising only a few minutes a day and you'll look like a supermodel are shortcuts that lead to failure. Realize that nothing of great significance is achieved without hard work. When talking about exercise, there is nothing truer than this. I get so frustrated when I see these hard-bodied models being spokespeople for exercise equipment they don't even use. The manufacturer leads you to believe that you can look like them by exercising on their equipment only a few minutes a day.

Dr. Cedric Bryant, Ph.D., chief exercise physiologist and vice president of educational services for the American Council on Exercise, says, "Infomercial claims are frequently overblown and some products are not very safe or effective." Furthermore, according to consumer reports, few if any infomercial products live up to their claim.

Or it's one of the hundreds of infomercials claiming their "diet pill" is the best. Who are these people trying to kid? Sure, you may see initial results and possibly lose some weight. But truthfully, are you going to stay on pills or an incredibly strict diet the rest of your life? No! How long can you really stand to eat grapefruits and water? There is no substitute for healthy nutritional choices that last a lifetime.

Part of the problem we face is that everybody is in a rush. We live in a "now" society. Nobody can wait. As a result people succumb to these "get in shape fast" propositions.

> "There are no shortcuts to any place worth going."
> ~ Beverly Sills

Taking shortcuts in your exercise program will never pay off. Beverly Sills was right when she said, "There are no shortcuts to any place worth going." You need to make time for your exercise program by making it a priority in your life.

In Chapter 6, "I Don't Have Time To Exercise," we'll look at just how much time you have available each day and how making exercise a priority in your life can benefit you. The chapter will conclude with six practical ways you can make room for exercise.

Finally, once you realize that succeeding with exercise isn't a series of shortcuts, but rather a lesson in perseverance, you'll be on your way to making exercise a part of your life. In the final chapter, "Persevere and Become Successful," we'll look at four ways to help you keep exercising and finish with how doing this will help you become successful in your life.

Failure Isn't Such a Bad Thing

Did any of those barriers ring a bell? Have you failed in one or more of those areas? Chances are you did. If so, don't worry...that's where this book will help.

Before we begin our journey toward making exercise a part of your life, I want to make something very clear. Just because you may have failed with exercise before doesn't mean you should never try again. In fact, many times, failure is a good thing.

Throughout history you can read about men and women who failed over and over before they became successful. What separates the successful from the failures is that they pick up the pieces and try again. Elbert Hubbard said, "Failure comes to a man who has blundered but wasn't able to cash in on the experience." On the same note, Dr. Ronald Niednagel says, "Failure isn't failure unless you don't learn from it." View it in this light and you will overcome obstacles.

Maybe you failed at exercise because you didn't see any results and quit. This may have occurred because you didn't really know how to put together an effective exercise program. Maybe you couldn't motivate yourself. Or, possibly, you had problems finding time to exercise that resulted in inconsistency, ultimately leading to your giving up.

If failure has been a part of your life, especially when it comes to exercise, don't despair. You can't take it personally. Appreciate failure and view it as a learning experience. As you read this book you'll learn what caused you to fail at exercise. But, be happy in the fact that you did fail because those failures have directed you toward the information necessary to becoming a success.

Making exercise work in your life is not something to be viewed as short-term. You have a lifetime to perfect it. There will be bumps, detours, and accidents on the road to exercise success. That last thing you ever want to do is give up!

Let's Get Started

Whether you've started an exercise program and failed, or never gotten started at all, this book is for you. Read it with a positive attitude and make a strong effort to apply the principles I teach. If you do, I'm certain you'll be inspired and well on your way to overcoming the obstacles that have held you back from making exercise a part of your life.

Walt Disney put it best when he said, "The way to get started is to quit talking and begin doing." This is great advice. Get started today!

CHAPTER 3

I Don't Know Where to Exercise

A Look at Your Options and
Who Can Help

"The great thing in this world is not so much where we are but in what direction we are moving."
~ Oliver Wendell Holmes

When a person finally makes the decision to start exercising, the first question that comes to mind is "Where am I going to work out?" There are several options available. Those include joining a health club, purchasing a home gym or exercising outside.

I'm going to focus on the choice of either joining a health club or purchasing a home gym. I believe that choosing one of these two options will give the best workout possible.

Although being outside sounds very inviting, it limits the workout to only certain types of exercises, therefore limiting the benefits you receive. When you exercise outside you are limited to cardiovascular exercise along with flexibility training. Outdoor exercise is not typically associated with strength training. Although cardiovascular exercise and flexibility training are very important, they should not be your only types of exercise. Strength training is a very important component and should not be neglected.

You may ask, "What about activities that involve lifting such as cutting wood, some types of landscaping or lifting bags of leaves or brush?" Technically you are lifting weight that involve muscular activity; however, it's not considered effective strength training. The reason is this. In order to strength train properly you must use each of the major muscle groups in a repetitive and consistent manner. This will create balance within each muscle group. Performing certain lifts such as stacking wood will only work certain muscle groups, leaving others virtually unused. Over time this may lead to muscular imbalance, later resulting in injury.

With that said, let's spend some time focusing on what you should know about joining a health club or purchasing a home gym.

Purchasing a Home Gym

You may decide to purchase a home gym for many different reasons.

Some people say that it's convenient to work out in their home. You don't have to worry about driving to the local health club. If the weather is bad, who cares, you don't have to leave home to work out.

For some it's a matter of self-consciousness. They would rather jump off a tall building than be seen in a health club.

Many times parents of small children don't want to go through the hassle of finding a babysitter while they work out, or they just don't want to pay for one. By having a home gym this eliminates the hassle.

People who spend a lot of time working find it hard to leave the office for exercise. As a result, they consider a home gym.

Finally, there are people who can get to the health club; however, don't feel like waiting in line for a machine or paying recurring membership dues.

Do any of these reasons sound familiar? If you answered "yes," I'll give you some guidelines to think about when purchasing a home gym. Keep in mind, however, having a home gym is great only if you are motivated to use it.

I've heard many stories of people who now belong to health clubs because they couldn't motivate themselves to get off the couch or out of bed to start exercising. Then you know what happens next. Their nice, expensive home gym becomes a haven for household spiders and their webs. Or maybe they don't want the gym to completely go to waste so it gets used as a clothes rack. Any clothes racks in your basement?

If you are confident this won't happen to you, then read on.

I've identified four factors you need to think about before purchasing home gym equipment.

Let's take a look at each one individually.

1. What are your needs?

The equipment should suit your needs and fitness level. It's important to ask yourself, "What do I want to accomplish?" It may be improvement of your cardiovascular system, more strength in your upper body or to increase your flexibility. Based on this you can determine the equipment that is best for you.

For the best results you should include equipment for strength, flexibility and cardiovascular training.

Strength training equipment

Strength training equipment can come in the form of multi-station machines, free weights or bands and tubing.

- Multi-station machines, sometimes called universal machines, combine several weight training stations into one frame. They offer a variety of strength training exercises all in one. Just a side note: make sure you can adjust the resistance on the machine. Being able to increase the resistance is important to ensure continuous results.

- Free weights are among the most common forms of home gym equipment. Free weights typically include dumbbells, a barbell with additional weights that can be added for more resistance, and some type of bench.

- Bands or tubing are the simplest form of strength training equipment. They are made from an elastic material that provides resistance when stretched. There are a number of strength training exercises that can be performed with these simple pieces of equipment. Also, they come in several different resistance levels.

Flexibility equipment

For flexibility training a simple mat will be sufficient. Even a mat isn't necessary if you have a carpeted floor. Also popular are cloth or nylon straps that aid you in your ability to stretch. They assist you in pulling the muscle through its full range of motion.

Cardiovascular equipment

When choosing cardiovascular equipment you have many options. They include treadmills, bikes, stair climbers, rowing machines, ski machines, elliptical trainers and more. The piece of equipment you choose is up to you. Choose one that you and the whole family will enjoy. You also need to ask yourself whether the particular piece of equipment is appropriate for you. What I mean by that is this: If you've had several knee surgeries, then a treadmill may not be your best option due to the impact and continuous pounding your joints endure. In this example, a bike may be the best choice, because there is no impact. Whatever the case, make sure you choose something you enjoy and are challenged by.

2. How much can you spend?

One rule that seems to hold true for many items is "you get what you pay for." I truly believe in this. If you purchase a cheaply priced treadmill, cheap is exactly what you will get. Keep in mind that high quality equipment usually can't be manufactured for a cheap price.

If you find yourself on a budget then you can always buy something like resistance bands, aerobic tapes or some light dumbbells. You are better off starting out with simple items such as these rather than buying a cheap piece of equipment that may fall apart, or worse, get you injured.

The opportunity is always there to purchase used equipment. Make sure to test it out, or better yet, go online and do some research on the exact make and model to see if it is a quality piece of equipment. In regards to exercise equipment, the American Council on Exercise, one of the leading exercise certification organizations in the country, encourages you to "try it out before you buy, especially when a significant financial investment is at stake."

At one point in my career I decided to put together a personal training studio in my finished basement. It was an ideal solution because we never used the basement and it had a lot of square footage to work with. At the time one of the clients I was training at the local gym told me she had a multi-station weight machine that she never used. Seeing this as a great opportunity, I thoroughly looked it over and took the time to test it out. In my opinion it checked out well. It turned out I had good judgment and the machine worked perfectly for the use I intended it. The best part about it is that I traded the woman personal training sessions for it, so it didn't cost me a dime.

If you look hard enough there is a good chance you will find the right piece of equipment. But, be careful you don't buy on impulse simply because you are anxious to get started. Do your homework!

3. Where will the equipment go?

Deciding where you want to put the equipment is really important. It has to be in a place where you will be motivated to work out. How motivated do you think you will be if you put it in a dark, dingy basement with no windows or nothing to look at? I'm guessing it won't be long before it gathers its share of cobwebs.

When deciding where the equipment should go, the most important factor to consider is safety. Here are some things to think about when choosing a location for your home gym.

- The area should be free of clutter.

- The floor should be solid, especially if you are setting up an area for lifting weights. It might be best to avoid weights in an upstairs room.

- You should have good lighting along with sufficient airflow. A room with a window is great because it provides light and airflow. If you don't have a window to open, then consider a fan.

- It is important to have an electrical outlet in the area to supply power to your equipment, a radio or additional lighting.

- Plan to have as much open space in the area as that taken up by equipment. This will give you room to maneuver.

To give you an idea on how much space to allow for various types of equipment, here are some general guidelines.

Treadmills—25-30 square feet

Bikes—10-15 square feet

Climber/stepper—15 square feet

Multi-station gym—50+ square feet

Free weights—30-50+ square feet

4. What are the product features?

This is a very important step that you don't want to miss. Not taking the time to look at the product features may lead to frustration, lack of use and wasted money. Let's look at features you need to consider when choosing home gym equipment.

- The machine should be comfortable for you. It should move in a manner that puts your body through the correct range of motion, thus ensuring safety. Unfortunately, most people (and maybe you're one of them) don't know what correct range of motion feels like. If you are buying from a dealer, then have the salesperson demonstrate and explain how their piece of equipment provides the correct range of motion. If you buy used equipment, then get on the machine and try it out. If it feels comfortable when going through each movement, chances are it will be fine.

- Another great feature to look for is the ability for the machine to adjust. Adjustments can come in the form of a moveable seat on a multi-station weight machine or bike, or speed and incline adjustments on a treadmill.

- Look for features that enhance safety. These may include guards on the weight stack or safety on/off switches on a treadmill.

- For many people, using a home gym will be a new experience. Having equipment that is easy to learn will make the experience more enjoyable.

- Finally, try to buy something that has a warranty. Nothing is worse than waiting to get your first piece of equipment only to have it break down in a month and cost you a mint to fix. Another advantage to a warranty is for maintenance purposes. Maintenance can be very expensive!

Not too long ago I had a conversation with a friend who purchased a treadmill for his home. He has owned the treadmill for approximately nine years now. He was telling me that over the years he has had the maintenance person come out to make various repairs. Just recently, something on the machine went wrong and ended up costing over $400 to repair. Thankfully he had continued to renew his warranty on the treadmill over the years and the repair cost him nothing. He estimated that he would have paid well over $1,000 in repair work since the time of purchase had he not kept extending the warranty. Definitely something to consider!

With the introduction of new home gym equipment, not to mention affordability, having a home gym is becoming very popular. It can be a great way to finally get started with that exercise program you have been talking about.

Take the time to consider the ideas I just listed before you buy any equipment. I have spoken with many people over the years who had the grand idea to build a home gym but later regretted it because it wasn't the right equipment or they just couldn't motivate themselves to work out on their own.

If you don't think a home gym is the best way for you to get started with exercise, then let's look at another possibility.

Joining a Health Club

As an owner/manager of a health club for over five years and another nine years of working at various health clubs, my advice will come with great value.

Health clubs today reach over 36 million people. A majority of these people are between the ages of 35 to 55 with the female population making up just over half of this total.

Believe it or not only 14% of the United States population belongs to a health club. I've always been amazed at how few people take advantage of the great opportunity a health club can offer. I think that many people are intimidated to join because a health club often gets stereotyped as a place where the young, perfectly shaped bodies get together to flaunt what they've got.

> ## Quick Fact
>
> **Health club members are more likely than others to report successful weight loss.**
> **~IHRSA Trend Report**

This is far from the truth. In fact, between 1987 and 2000, health club membership for Americans over the age of 55 grew 350%, according to the International Health, Racquet and Sportsclub Association (IHRSA) in Boston. This means that nearly one out of every five club members today is over the age of 55.

Joining a health club can be one of the most rewarding decisions you ever make. Before you spend any money joining a health club, look at the following suggestions I have to find one that best fits your needs.

There are three important areas to consider when choosing a health club: personal preparation before joining, what to look for and making the best use of the club.

1. Personal preparation before joining

As a person who has sold thousands of health club member-ships over the years, I can't emphasize enough how important it is to identify your fitness goals before walking into a health club for the first time. So many people walk in to a club and have no idea what type of questions to ask. Their question is usually "How much does it cost?"

Every membership salesperson cringes when this question is asked first. As a prospective member you have to know what the club has to offer and how it can benefit you before asking the price. What if the price, if asked first, seems too high? You may walk out of the club, go down the street and join the club that is priced lower. Only after you've made a commitment to the cheaper club do you realize it was a big mistake. The club you joined, because it was cheaper, isn't able to meet your needs. Or worse yet, the staff is unfriendly and unwilling to help. Now you're stuck!

The point I'm trying to make is that if you know what your needs and goals are, then you can ask questions that help determine if the club can meet those needs.

Now, although I did say that cost should not be your first consideration, it is an important factor. Take a look at your budget and determine the maximum amount you can afford on a monthly basis. By doing this you will be better equipped to make a

> **Know what your needs and goals are, then ask questions accordingly.**

decision about joining the day you walk in the club. The sales staff will love you for it.

I can tell you of countless people who say they have to think about it because they don't take the time to figure out before-hand what they really want and can afford. Unfortunately, many people who say they need to think about it never come back. And worse yet, they never start an exercise program at all. Don't let this be you. Prepare!

2. What to look for

There are many things to consider when looking for a health club that will meet your needs. Following are some of what I think are the most important ones to consider.

In order to make as informed a decision as possible, I recommend setting up a tour of the club with one of the membership staff. Ask a lot of questions during the tour. Not only will the salesperson enjoy it, but also you will learn everything you need to know about the club.

The following are some characteristics of the club you need to familiarize yourself with. Use these as an outline for questions to ask on your tour.

Qualifications of the staff

This is one of the most important features to look for in a club. It's unfortunate, but this day and age anyone can call themselves a personal trainer. You don't need a license or certification to be one. However, a certification is highly recommended (more on this later). If you are unfortunate enough to get a trainer with no background education or worse yet, little experience, you will get frustrated. The frustration may come from lack of results or injury due to improper form. I really believe that anyone who calls themselves a personal trainer should be certified from an accredited organization. Later in this chapter I will discuss in more detail what you should look for in a personal trainer.

Friendliness of the staff

The biggest fear people have when joining a club is not feeling comfortable. A good staff will welcome you with open arms. You should be greeted by first name and with a smile each time you walk in the building. The staff should be helpful, knowledgeable, and courteous.

My staff is required to walk the floor and offer help and encouragement to the members on a daily basis. I let them know at every staff meeting that this is crucial if they want to keep their jobs. As a result, our reputation in the community is based on a staff that gets to know each member by name and is always willing to offer assistance.

Hours of operation

Health clubs across the country vary greatly in the hours they are open. Make sure that the club's hours of operation fit your schedule. Nothing is worse than joining a club and later realizing that they are closed during the time you prefer to work out.

Cleanliness and good maintenance

This is self-explanatory. Walking into a locker room with mold growing in the corners isn't what most people prefer. Ask questions regarding the cleaning schedule. When looking at the fitness floor, do you see "out of order" signs on various machines? If you do, it may be a sign of neglect. Another absolute "no-no" for a heath club is when duct tape is used to hold things together. This type of environment will not make for a good exercise experience.

Crowdedness

The best way to determine whether or not you will have to wait for a machine is to tour the club at the time you will most likely be using it. If it is jam-packed at the time you walk in that day, then chances are it's the same way every day. Now, there is an exception. You'll find that Mondays are more crowded than any other day of the week. I think Mondays are busy because many people have a little too much fun on the weekends. Could that be you, perhaps?

Amenities

There are many different types of amenities health clubs offer. Some examples include aerobics or Pilates classes, a juice bar, a pro shop, tanning, spa treatments, basketball or other court sports, towel service, Internet access on the cardiovascular equipment, sauna, hot tub, pool and many others. You need to decide what amenities fit your needs and use that in your decision whether or not to join.

I highly recommend shopping around. Go and see what each club in your area has to offer. Many clubs will have a free trial membership. Some may give you one day while others may allow you to try it for two weeks. I've even heard of clubs offering 30 days free. Take advantage of these free trial memberships in order to make the right decision.

Location

Choosing a club that is close to your home or workplace is critical in determining your success. You are more likely to use the club if it is in a convenient location. However, don't choose a club just for this reason. It must meet your needs.

3. Making the best use of the club

Joining the club of your choice is just the beginning. Once you've joined you need to make good use of it.

A great way to get started is to immediately make an appointment with a personal trainer.

A good trainer will talk to you about your goals and health history. Based on this he or she will design a training program customized to your needs followed by a full demonstration of all the exercises. In most clubs there is no additional fee for this service.

Look into the schedule of aerobic or other group training classes. Find out if there are any that interest you. If there are, then try them out. A group setting is motivational and can be very invigorating.

> "The way to get started is to quit talking and begin doing."
> ~Walt Disney

Remember to exercise at your own pace. Don't worry about what others are doing. You don't have to impress anyone but yourself.

Finally, make sure the club offers a variety of exercises. Boredom can set in quickly with the same ole monotonous routine. The trainers at the club can be very helpful at suggesting a variety of exercises for your workout.

Understanding a Membership Contract

Before we leave our discussion on choosing a health club, it's important to mention the membership contract. One of the most frustrating issues a health club manager has to face is with people who don't understand the membership papers they've just signed.

Membership contracts can come in various forms. You need to understand what type of membership you are buying. Is it a multi-year contract, an annual membership, or a month-to-month agreement? Generally you will get a different price per month depending on the length of term. Know what you are getting into.

I can't tell you how many people I have dealt with over the years that call me after several months and say they want to cancel their membership. That's fine if the membership is set to expire; however, many of them want to cancel in the middle of their contract. When I tell them they still have a given number of months remaining on their contract they get defensive and tell me they didn't remember signing anything that says they are obligated to a certain number of months. It's an easy argument for me; all I do is pull out the membership agreement and show them what they signed.

> **Read the membership contract and know what you are signing.**

Also, I would suggest you ask the club if there are any circumstances that would allow you to get out of a contract if necessary. Some examples may include when you move out of town or if you develop a medical condition that prohibits you from using the club.

It all boils down to reading the membership contract and asking questions if there is something you don't understand before you sign it! And yes, that means reading the fine print. Neglecting this may come back to haunt you someday.

Final Words on
Joining a Health Club

You may say my opinion is biased because I manage a health club, but joining one is the best and safest way to begin an exercise program. The availability of a knowledgeable and educated staff will go a long way in making your exercise experience a positive one. In addition, the social atmosphere alone is very motivating and encouraging for most people.

Don't believe the myth that health clubs are full of people who are young and in great shape. The truth is they are filled with people just like you, ranging in age from teenagers to those in their 90s. Everybody is there to get in shape, not to pick on you.

Should I Hire a Personal Trainer?

Personal training has existed for close to 20 years in the United States. Originally it started out for actors and actresses being trained for their roles in the movies and to keep in top physical condition. They made up the majority of the clientele because they were the only ones who could afford it.

While at one time personal training may have been limited to the wealthy, more and more it is becoming less exclusive.

According to a survey conducted by American Sports Data, there are more than 88,000 personal trainers that work with over 5.6 million Americans each year.

Why are so many people choosing to hire personal trainers? Because they realize the results attained with a personal trainer can be far superior to what they can do on their own. Trainers make this possible by creating individualized and specific exercise prescriptions. When you throw this together with a powerful motivator and expert guidance, it spells success.

> ### Quick Fact
> ___
> Over 5.6 million people use the services of a personal trainer.

Clients put a lot of trust in the trainer and expect results superior to what they can accomplish on their own. The last thing a client wants is to throw away a bunch of money on a trainer who isn't knowledgeable and can't motivate.

To get the most from a trainer and your workout, make sure you hire one that has experience, is educated and possesses the attributes necessary to help you be successful. Before you hire a personal trainer, consider the following characteristics.

1. Technical knowledge and certification

The educational level of personal trainers can range from what they learn on their own to having a doctorate degree in exercise physiology. Currently, there are no federal or state laws that say who can or cannot practice as a personal trainer. This leaves the door wide open for anyone to call themselves a personal trainer.

There are approximately 400 personal training certifications offered today; however, only six have risen to prominence. They include certifications from the American Council on Exercise (ACE), the American College of Sports Medicine (ACSM), the Aerobics and Fitness Association of America (AFAA), the National Academy of Sports Medicine (NASM), the National Strength and Conditioning Association (NSCA), and the Young Men's Christian Association (YMCA).

Trainers with one of these certifications will set themselves apart from the others. Furthermore, it is important for trainers to continuously educate themselves in order to stay up-to-date with the latest training technologies. It is for this reason

> **F.Y.I.**
>
> **Of over 400 certifications, fewer than six require minimum standards.**

that many of the credible certifying organizations require continuing education units to keep the certification current.

When choosing a personal trainer I would highly recommend you ask about each trainer's credentials and certification. It may mean the difference between seeing results and wasting your money.

2. *Educational background*

More and more personal trainers are seeking a degree in exercise science or other related field. Those that really want to set themselves apart will have a bachelor's or master's degree in their field. This type of background provides the trainer with a deep knowledge of anatomy, physiology, kinesiology (movement), and technical skill.

What does this mean to you the client? It means safer lifting technique, more comfortable movement patterns and a more effective workout. I must point out, however, the trainer must be able to take this knowledge and apply it to the client in order to see positive changes. This is where the next point becomes important.

3. *Experience*

Although I think that technical knowledge and educational background are extremely important factors in choosing a personal trainer, experience cannot be overlooked. A trainer with good experience is one who has had a number of clients over a period of time. There is no substitute for practical training experience.

A trainer's experience will tell you if he or she has a proven track record. After all, you don't want to hire a trainer that isn't providing results. Looking at their experience may also tell you the type of clients they feel comfortable with. For example, the trainer may be more interested in working with athletes than those seeking weight loss. Find a trainer that has experience working with people who have the same needs as you.

4. *Communication skills and a talkative nature*

Here is something for you to think about. You hire a trainer to help you lose 15 pounds before your vacation in four months. You go down to the local health club and ask for the names of some personal trainers. So they give you a name and number of the trainer to call. Being a busy person you decide to e-mail him. He responds quickly and immediately gives you information on his educational background, certification and experience with other clients. You think, "this guy seems like he knows what he is doing. I think I'll hire him." So you send a check and set up the first training appointment.

During the first appointment he asks you about your health history and goals, then suggests a body fat test and circumference measurements. Upon leaving the appointment, you feel really good.

But that is where the positive results end.

At your next appointment, your first real training appointment, he begins by putting you through the workout he designed. The workout seems fine; however, the trainer is very quiet. Twenty minutes into the session he hasn't said a whole lot. In fact, all he does is count out loud the repetitions you are performing. Ten–nine–eight–seven–six and on and on. Once in a while he throws in a "good job, one more rep." During the session you try to strike up a conversation with him, but to no avail.

"The next exercise works your triceps...let's get started," he says.

Unsure about how he wants you to perform the exercise, you ask him to explain it to you. "Grasp the handle like this and push it down!" he exclaims as he demonstrates, using an imaginary handle.

By the end of the workout you are bored out of your mind and unmotivated. He has never made eye contact with you and many times while you were performing an exercise, he was looking at someone else across the room.

You say to yourself, "on paper this guy looked like he was a great trainer." What you couldn't tell from the e-mail was that he was a poor communicator. Later you find out the experience he mentioned was with several other clients like yourself, that only lasted a few sessions due to boredom.

> **Take the time to meet with your prospective personal trainer in person.**

If you are going to hire a personal trainer, be sure to meet this person one on one before you sign a contract. A great personal trainer is one that knows how to communicate. They must be a talker.

You as the client will have many questions that need to be thoroughly answered. The trainer needs to deliver. He should describe and demonstrate the exercises in detail as well as explain why you are doing each exercise.

Beyond having communication skills, a trainer needs to be motivating. It's hard for a silent person to be very motivating. The trainer needs to get you fired up. They need to get you excited and make you want to be there. This is what produces results and makes you want to go back for more.

5. Creativity

The last important attribute is the trainer's ability to build a creative program. Any trainer can put together an exercise program. You need to find one who knows the importance of variety.

At first any program will provide interest and results; however, that may only last for a short period of time. At some point the trainer will need to identify whether or not the program is still producing results and enthusiasm. When a new program is put together, it should be interesting and creative. The longer you exercise, the more creativity is necessary.

If possible, ask some of the personal trainer's clients how creative he or she is. Who better to ask? If the trainer is always providing them with something new and interesting then you can be sure the same will probably hold true for you. Seek out a creative trainer—you won't regret it.

There are many other attributes that make up a great personal trainer, such as honesty, integrity, concern for people, a positive attitude, and a fit physique as evidence that they regularly train themselves.

My best advice to you is that you meet with the trainer, look at their qualifications, get a chance to talk in person and, lastly, go with your gut instinct.

Begin by Getting Started

One of the hardest things for people to do when deciding to exercise is to get started. The greatest intent isn't worth anything when you can't get started.

Whether you decide to exercise outside, at home, or in a health club, you need to take action. Just thinking about it won't help you lose weight. Theodore Hesburgh once said, "My basic principle is that you don't make decisions because they are easy; you don't make them because they're cheap; you don't make them because they're popular; you make them because they're right."

The right decision isn't going to come in just deciding where to exercise. The right decision will be made when you decide that this is the day I'm going to start exercising.

Review this chapter and determine what will be best for you. Once you know, don't hesitate to get started.

CHAPTER 4

I Don't Know How to Exercise

What You Need to Know
In Order to Get Started

*"The more I learn the more I realize I don't know, and
the more I realize I don't know the more I want to
learn."*
~ *Albert Einstein*

When you think of exercise, what is the first thing that comes to mind? Is it walking or jogging, maybe taking a bike ride or following an aerobics tape? If this is what you are thinking, you are partially correct.

Exercise should consist of three parts: cardiovascular (aerobic) training, strength training, and flexibility training. It is very important to include all three of these components in your program. Many people associate exercise with just cardiovascular activity—that includes activities such as walking, biking, jogging, and aerobic tapes along with many others. For some, doing work around the house is thought of as exercise. Although you may sweat a little or really feel like you've done something, it isn't a well-rounded exercise program. An effective exercise program must include all three components. Let's take a look.

Cardiovascular Training

Most likely you've participated in some type of cardiovascular training. If you ever went for a walk, rode a bike, ran a race, paddled a canoe, cross-country skied, or played a recreational sport, then you have participated in cardiovascular exercise. And this just names a few activities.

Why is cardiovascular training so important for the body? Because it maintains the health of the most important muscle in your body...your heart. Cardiovascular training is responsible for improving blood pressure, cholesterol, and circulation, all this leading to a lower risk of heart disease. In addition it can reduce anxiety levels, give you more energy to meet the demands of daily life, and allow you to consume greater quantities of food and still maintain caloric balance.

Let's Look at the Options

In the previous chapter we discussed your options regarding where to exercise. Your decision whether you chose to exercise at home or at a health club will determine which of the following exercises are best for you.

Outdoor cardiovascular exercise

If you prefer to exercise on your own and would like to spend time outside, there are many activities to choose from. You can enjoy exercises such as biking, walking, jogging, running, swimming, canoeing, kayaking, rowing a boat, hiking, cross-country skiing, snowshoeing, and ice skating. Weather permitting these are all great choices. I'll bet you can think of others.

Indoor cardiovascular exercises

If you choose to exercise indoors and have your own equipment or belong to a health club, you can use a treadmill, bike, rower, stairstepper, elliptical trainer, airdyne or one of the many other types of indoor equipment available today. If you don't have access to equipment or need to be inside, try jumping rope, jogging or marching in place, performing jumping jacks or working out to aerobic tapes. It is important that

---

Training Tip

Finding something you enjoy will establish a lasting habit.

you select a type of exercise you find enjoyable. Finding something you enjoy will establish a lasting habit. When you find something enjoyable, don't let this be your one and only source of cardiovascular exercise...mix it up!! You don't want it to get boring and monotonous.

Don't Forget to Monitor Your Heart Rate

An often-neglected component of cardiovascular exercise is the knowledge of where your heart rate is during the training session. How many times have you gone for a walk around your neighborhood without checking your heart rate? This happens often. Although there is nothing wrong with it, you may not get the results you are capable of producing. Here's why. Since walking is so common to us (we do it every day), our heart isn't really stimulated by the activity. What you need to do is know where your heart rate is at during the walk (or any other physical activity for that matter) to achieve beneficial results.

What should your heart rate be? Let's look at a simple formula for figuring this out.

Target Heart Rate = (220 - AGE) X .60 to .90

This is a simple formula for determining target heart rate; however, there are others that take into account other variables. Generally speaking, this formula is used most often for simplicity's sake. The number "220" represents, hypothetically, the maximum a heart can beat. In order to customize this formula you subtract your age from 220, giving you the maximum your heart can beat in one minute. The .60 and .90 represent a percentage of the maximum your heart can beat.

For example, if you are 40 years old, subtract 40 from 220, for a figure of 180. 180 x .60 = 108 beats per minute, or the minimum for your cardiovascular benefit; 180 x .90 = 162 beats per minute, or the maximum for you.

The higher the percentage the more intensely you are working out. This higher intensity, if it is above the intensity you normally work out at, will force your body to change in order to adapt to the new stimulus. This change is normally positive.

It is important that you monitor your heart rate at various times throughout your cardiovascular activity, in order to achieve maximum results. You can monitor your heart rate by finding your pulse. Use a watch or clock with a second

hand. Count for 6 seconds and multiply that number by 10; or count for 10 seconds and multiply that number by 6. Or use a heart rate monitor. Heart rate monitors can be purchased at stores that sell sporting goods or you can buy one online. They come in a variety of models, each one with a different set of bells and whistles. A standard model, measuring only heart rate, works just fine.

How High Should I Have My Heart Rate?

Over the years you may have heard or read that if you work out at a lower intensity (say 60 to 70% of maximum heart rate) then you are more likely to burn body fat. On the other hand, working out at a higher intensity (70 to 90% of maximum heart rate) will improve cardiovascular fitness, meaning more stamina and improved cardiac functioning. To some degree this is true.

A lower intensity tends to utilize fat as your energy source, so you may burn more body fat while working out at a lower heart rate. However, you'll need to exercise for a longer period of time. Keep in mind, the formula for losing weight is simple...expend

more calories than you consume. So whether you exercise at a low intensity or a high intensity, what matters is the total number of calories you burn during the exercise session. If you choose to exercise at a lower heart rate you will need to increase the duration of your workout in order to burn more calories.

If you think about it, the best heart rate to work out at is at a higher percentage of your maximum. Not only are you burning more calories, but you're also training at an intensity that is more conducive for improving cardiac function.

I want to point out a cautionary note regarding the intensity of your workout. A higher intensity may burn more calories in a shorter period of time along with greater conditioning of the heart; however, you need to be the judge whether or not you can handle it. If you're feeling faint, lightheaded or dizzy, that's a sign you're overdoing it. Ease up and slowly increase the intensity over time. Don't ignore the warning signs your body gives you. Again, make sure you check with your doctor before beginning an exercise program.

Recommendations for Cardiovascular Training

The American College of Sports Medicine recommends you train your cardiovascular system every other day for 30 to 40 minutes. The American Heart Association recommends 30 minutes daily. The Centers for Disease Control and Prevention suggests at least 30 minutes of moderate physical activity most days. Studies have shown that even spending 10 minutes at three separate times a day can make a difference. So if you can't find 30 minutes in one block of time, then try several bouts of 10 minutes.

The fact of the matter is that anything is better than nothing. People have achieved nice results spending 20 minutes three times a week. You ask, "Can I do more?" Absolutely! By doing more you will be able to burn more calories and possibly see greater improvement in the efficiency of your heart and lungs. However, remember, more isn't always better. Listen to your body. If you feel worn out all the time or find yourself not looking forward to exercise, that may be a sign you are overtraining. If this is the case, cut back and allow your body to recover.

I've worked with many people in the past who feel that if they aren't seeing progress, they need to do more. This will often lead to burnout or injury, therefore really halting progress. Take my word for it, more is not always better and it doesn't hurt to take a couple days off here and there.

Strength Training

In the past, strength training was viewed as something that only men participate in. You've probably seen pictures or video clips of men standing around a bench press yelling and screaming with sweat pouring out of their skin trying to lift a little more weight than the guys next to them.

Those days are over. Men and women alike are getting involved with strength training due to the incredible benefits it provides. In fact, according to a study in 2001 by American Sports Data, Inc., women accounted for 45% of all those who strength train using free weights. This number is up from 30% in 1987.

So, whether you want to build muscle or just want to tone up, strength training plays a vital role.

Strength training plays host to many great changes in the body. The most obvious is the increase in muscle strength and, if enough effort is applied, muscle size. Some of the not-so-obvious results include increased bone density, improved tendon and ligament strength, improved joint function, increased muscular endurance, and many more.

Fitness Fact

Women account for 45% of all those who strength train using free weights.

I want to mention something that is often a fear for women who are contemplating starting a strength training program. That is the fear of developing big, bulky muscles. Building muscle is not easy. It is especially difficult for women because they are lacking in an essential muscle-building hormone called testosterone. Women should look toward strength training for another very important reason...increasing bone density. Osteoporosis is a real issue. Eighty percent of those who get osteoporosis are women. One in two women will have an osteoporosis-related fracture at some point in her life. Strength training is a way you can help prevent this disease that is quickly becoming a major public health threat.

A Secret About Strength Training

Strength training can actually increase your metabolism! Your metabolism is the rate at which your body burns fat. Simply put, the higher your metabolism the more body fat you will be able to burn during daily activities and at rest.

You probably know a person who, no matter what he or she eats, never seems to put on an ounce of fat. These people disgust you, right? People like this are probably blessed with a naturally high metabolism, allowing them to indulge while not having to worry about gaining a pound.

You're probably thinking, "Good for them, what about me?" You're in luck. Strength training is the ticket, among other things, to increasing your metabolism.

Remember, the higher your metabolism, the more body fat and calories you'll burn. Now that you see the benefits strength training can provide, let's take a look at how you can get started.

Forms of Strength Training Available

Strength training comes in several forms: body weight exercises, circuit machines, free weights, and through the use of bands and tubing. Again, your decision on where to work out will impact what type of equipment you use.

1. Bodyweight strength training exercises

Body weight exercises are strength-training exercises that use only your body weight. They are not as effective as other forms of strength training. However, if it is your only means, they can be beneficial. Some of the most common body weight strength training exercises include squats, lunges, push-ups, sit-ups, pull-ups, and calf raises.

As you may notice, I didn't include pictures demonstrating the strength training exercises in this book. I feel that, although pictures may be helpful, they don't effectively teach you the proper mechanics of the exercise. I highly recommend you hire a personal trainer or visit your local health club and seek professional instruction for any strength training exercises you begin.

Although body weight exercises are a simple way to get started, because you don't need equipment, the limited number of exercises result in boredom and reaching a plateau rather quickly.

2. Home Gym or Health Club Strength Training Exercises

When you get to the point where body weight exercises become boring and no longer elicit results, the next logical step would be to purchase home gym equipment or join a health club. Both options provide a variety of exercises where you have the option to add weight to the exercise. Strength training exercises provided by a home gym or health club can take you to the next level in your strength training workout.

Our bodies are remarkable in their ability to adapt to the stimuli we place upon them. That is why it's important to make changes to your exercise program on a frequent basis. By utilizing more advanced equipment, the type you find in a home gym or health club, you can shock your body into changing for the better.

I've worked with a number of people over the years who spent most of their workout doing only cardiovascular exercise along with a few body weight strength training exercises. These people will often ask me why they haven't seen much progress despite consistently working out. I'll tell them they need to add a new element to their program, that element being strength training exercises using added weight. It usually doesn't take long and they come back to me saying that they are back to seeing results.

As a personal trainer, I like to change my client's programs every six to eight weeks. My clients enjoy exercise more because of the variety in the exercises. The variety of equipment in a home gym or health club makes it simple to do this.

3. *Free weight exercises*

The use of machines for strength training can be effective for a long period of time. Eventually, however, you will again want a change. The next change should be a move to free weights. Free weights offer even more variety than a home gym or circuit weight machines at a health club.

The use of free weights involves lifting weight with a dumbbell or barbell. Dumbbells are the single hand-held weights that can range from one to 200 lbs. A single dumbbell is held in each hand and lifted independently of the other. A barbell is a long bar that typically weighs 45 lbs and can be loaded with extra weight to increase the resistance. The barbell is lifted as a single unit.

At first, you may find strength training with free weights to be difficult because a great deal of balance and stability are required for a successful lift. Once you've learned the technique and the ability to balance and stabilize, you are at a great advantage. Here's why. The extra effort required to balance and stabilize the weights creates the need for more energy and muscular activation, therefore providing greater results. Results come in the form of more calories being burned, greater muscular development, and increased coordination.

Structuring Strength Training Exercises Into a Program

Now that you're schooled in the variety of strength training exercises available, let's look at how to put everything together into a program.

There is no one right program. We all have different needs, desires, goals and health histories that require analysis before an effective program is designed. For example, do you think the same training program would be given to a person who has had lower back surgery as for someone who is training to run a marathon? The answer is no! Programs need to be designed on an individual basis. Don't let anyone tell you otherwise.

I get frustrated when I hear about people following programs they get from magazines. What can be even more frustrating are the people writing them. People are led to believe that just because a program is found in a popular fitness magazine it will work for them. This is not always the case. People need to be careful what they start. I guess, in the writer's defense, these programs are written with the intent that people who decide to try them know whether or not they are capable of performing the exercises.

> ## Training Tip
>
> **A strength training program should be customized based on your health history, needs, and goals.**

Beware, just because a program is written by someone from a fitness magazine doesn't mean it will work for you. Be careful what you read make sure you are physically ready for it.

With that said, I'm going to make some suggestions for putting together a general strength training program you can try, providing you can answer yes to the following assumptions.

The first assumption is that you already know how to perform the particular exercises chosen. Second, that you have no history of injuries or ailments that require specific concern (i.e., surgeries, heart disease, diabetes, joint conditions, etc.). Finally, that you are looking to just get started with a strength-training program and have no real specific needs but to get in shape.

If you answered yes to all of these, then the following suggestions will be helpful to you. However, you must keep in mind that eventually changes will need to be made.

A strength-training program should consist of exercises that work each of the major muscle groups. These include shoulders, chest, back, arms, midsection and legs. A group of eight to 10 exercises will generally cover all the areas of the body. I would suggest that you perform two sets of eight to 12 repetitions for each exercise.

A repetition is, for example, one bicep curl or one leg press.

A set is a group of repetitions. If you perform two sets of eight to 12 repetitions you are actually lifting the weight 16 to 24 times with a short rest in the middle.

I would suggest a one-minute rest interval between sets. This will allow for adequate recovery.

A question I often get is, "Should I do eight or 12 repetitions? Why is there a range?" The range of repetitions is there to monitor progress. You want to pick a weight with which you can correctly complete at least eight repetitions but not more than 12. If you are able to perform more than 12 repetitions, you need to add more weight. It's very important that you try to increase weight as soon as performing 12 repetitions becomes easy for you.

What happens in this instance is that the body adapts to the stimulus and it doesn't see the need for change. You need to create a new stress as often as possible. It is the adaptation to the stress that creates the change you desire.

I would recommend you strength train three non-consecutive days per week. However, if you are still feeling sore and are scheduled for another workout, rest another day. Your body is telling you that you are not fully recovered. Listen to it! The biggest mistake people make is that they do too much. Believe in the power of rest. It's important.

> ## Training Tip
>
> ---
>
> **Change your exercise program every eight to 12 weeks to insure progress.**

Although I recommend strength training three non-consecutive days a week, this is not the only way to do it. If you train different muscle groups, it is acceptable to strength train on consecutive days. Individual needs and goals will determine what is best for you. As I mentioned earlier, adequate rest is important regardless of your training style.

Strength training is a valuable tool when trying to get in shape. It is great for people of all ages; however, caution must be taken depending on your age and health history. Take the time to learn how to perform strength-training exercises properly. It will save you a lot of time, frustration, and potential injury.

It's important to remember that the recommendations I made are very general. A program can be changed in many ways. Variety can be sought in the form of changing exercises, repetitions, sets, rest intervals, frequency, and duration of the repetition plus many more.

It's crucial to remember, when designing a strength training program, to look at your own individual needs and desires. Then you can design, or have a personal trainer design, a program best fit for you.

Flexibility Training

The third and final component of an exercise program is stretching to enhance your flexibility. This is the easiest part of your program. Many people, however, neglect this important component. It doesn't take very long and can even be mixed between sets in your strength training program.

Before you begin stretching it is important to get the body warmed up. Here is a great analogy describing why a warm-up is important.

Let's say you live in the northern part of the country and it is a cold winter day (a bone-chilling five below zero). Your newspaper has just been delivered to your mailbox at the end of the driveway. Excited to read the latest headline, you bundle up and run out to the mailbox. The newspaper is wrapped up in a rubber band to keep it intact. You grab the rubber band and quickly pull it off. When you pull at the ice-cold rubber band, what do you think is going to happen? Snap, it breaks off!

Let's replay this scenario and say that you aren't in a hurry to read the newspaper so you bring it into the house with the rubber band still wrapped around it. Five minutes later you decide to pull the rubber band off so you can read the paper. The house is a warm 75 degrees, so what do you think will happen to the rubber band? It stretches!

Although your muscles probably won't snap if you neglect your warm-up, you can see my point. Your chance of injury is less if you take a few minutes to warm up before stretching. You can do this by walking, jumping rope or any other easy activity to elevate your heart rate and body temperature.

The Flexibility Training Program

When stretching, as with strength training, it is important to work each of the major muscle groups. Again, that being the shoulders, chest, arms, midsection, back and legs.

I recommend you hold each stretch for 15 to 30 seconds. Is it bad to hold it longer? No, not at all, but some people find that holding it too long is boring. If it feels good and you really enjoy stretching, go ahead and hold each stretch a little longer. On the other hand, holding a stretch for only several seconds may not be adequate. I would rather err on the side of holding too long rather than too briefly.

While performing the stretch, make sure you feel it in the area you are targeting. It's very easy to go through the motions of stretching and not concentrate on what you are doing. It shouldn't be painful, but a good stretch may be slightly uncomfortable. In time, your flexibility will increase and you will need to reach a little further on your stretches.

> ### Fitness Fact
> ------
> **As we age our bodies tend to lose flexibility and become less mobile.**

A good stretching program may only take several minutes. Don't neglect this component of exercise because it seems insignificant. As we age our bodies tend to lose flexibility and become less mobile. Harvey Lauer, president of American Sports Data, Inc. says, "For many people, especially those over the age of 55, stretching is an important exercise in its own right." Making sure flexibility is a part of your program will be very beneficial as you get older.

Putting It All Together

There you have it, the basics of each component of fitness—cardiovascular, strength and flexibility training. You're probably asking, "How do I put all this together?" It's not as hard as you may think. It's important to remember that everybody is different and an exercise program can vary from person to person. Again, the following is a suggestion based on your answering yes to the previously mentioned assumptions. Here is what I suggest. It's best to perform the exercises in the order below.

Warm-up

- Spend three to five minutes warming up.

- The warm-up should consist of some light cardiovascular activity to slightly elevate your heart rate and body temperature.

- Also, this is the time I would suggest you do some flexibility exercises.

Strength training

- Perform eight to 10 different exercises making sure to involve each of the major muscle groups.

- For each exercise do two sets of eight to 12 repetitions.

- Allow one-minute rest intervals between sets and exercises.

- Strength train three non-consecutive days a week, for example on Monday, Wednesday, and Friday.

Cardiovascular training

- Train three to five days per week. This can be accomplished on days you weight train or on opposite days—whatever works best for you.

- It is okay to perform cardiovascular exercise on consecutive days.

- Know your target heart rate and work out in the range that is best suited to your goals and fitness level.

- It is best to train at least 30 minutes continuously, several days a week.

Cool-down

- Similarly to the warm-up, spend three to five minutes cooling down.

- Your cool-down can be an extension of the cardiovascular training exercise. Take a few extra minutes at a slower pace, allowing your heart rate to decrease to near pre-workout levels.

• This would again be a good time to do some more flexibility exercises. It may reduce some of the soreness for the next day.

Now It's Your Turn!

There is no question that exercise is difficult. Trying to design and utilize a program with little or no knowledge can be frustrating and time-consuming. It's good to know there are people who can help.

Over the years I've put together numerous programs for myself, some that worked well and some that didn't. There is a lot of trial and error involved, based on how our bodies respond to the exercise stimulus. Realize you need to find a program that works for you. One program will not fit all.

As mentioned earlier, many people look to popular fitness magazines for advice on how to exercise. Some of the programs suggested may be great for one person and not so great for the next. You must take into consideration your health history, needs, and goals. You will know fairly quickly if the program is working or not. Boredom, lack of enthusiasm, or a feeling that nothing is happening are sure signs you need to make a change in your program.

A program may only last you one month before you feel a change is necessary. On the other hand, it may last four months. As long as you continue to see and feel results with your current program, and are enthusiastic about it, then stick with it. Many times you are the best judge regarding the effectiveness of the program, not necessarily a fitness professional.

Take the advice written in this chapter and get started with an exercise program that includes each of the three exercise components. I encourage you to seek every opportunity to learn how you can improve your exercise program on a regular basis. Stretch your mind as you would your muscles!

CHAPTER 5

I'm too Inconsistent With Exercise

Five Steps to Making Exercise a Habit

"Habits are powerful factors in our lives. Because they are consistent, often unconscious patterns, they constantly, daily, express our character and produce our effectiveness...or ineffectiveness."

~ Steven R. Covey

It's December 31st and you are at a New Year's Eve party with all your friends. Suddenly, someone has the bright idea that everyone should share their New Year's resolutions.

Everyone gets in a circle and you begin to exchange resolutions. When it is your turn, you tell them you want to lose 20 lbs. and trim a couple inches off your waistline. Furthermore, you let them know you're planning on joining a health club so you can immediately get started.

The New Year arrives and you make your way down to the local health club and buy a membership. They are very helpful and quickly get you on an exercise program to begin your weight loss. Along with you are many other people with the same New Year's resolution.

For the first few weeks things are going well. You seem to feel like it's working and have already shaved off a couple pounds. "This is great," you say.

Unexpectedly, during the fourth week, you get buried at work with a project that has to be completed by week's end. As a result, you can't make it to the health club or even go for a walk outside the entire week.

Finally, you finish the project, but are mentally exhausted from all the late nights working on it. Another week passes before you think about getting to the club.

After a two-week layoff you make it back to the club and start your exercise program again. This layoff and the stress of the project cause you to lose a little strength and forget some of the exercises. So you ask one of the trainers who gladly helps. The problem is that you're irritated by the fact you already forgot some of the exercises and have lost strength.

Anticipating a little soreness from the exercise, because it's been two weeks since you last lifted weights, you decide to take the rest of the week off.

So, now it's into mid-February, you started off well, but have only exercised once in the last three weeks. And to make matters worse, you have a vacation planned for the end of the week and can't work out because you have to tie up some loose ends at work as well as pack for the trip.

Following your vacation you don't feel like having to re-learn the exercises and, physically, are right back where you on January 1st. As a result, you give up. The once grand resolution to lose some weight is over.

Great Intentions

I've been involved in the fitness industry for over 14 years and this story is nothing new. I have seen it played out year after year. Grand plans to get fit end up fizzling.

Has this ever happened to you? As you were reading the story did anything hit home? If you answered "yes" you are not alone.

Each year nearly 100 million Americans will make a New Year's resolution, the most common being health related. The sad thing is that only 40% of people will be successful on the first attempt.

> ### F.Y.I.
>
> **Each year nearly 100 million Americans will make a New Year's resolution, with the most common being health related.**

When you walk into a health club in January, it's amazing how busy it can be. The enthusiasm and excitement to make the resolution work is evident. However, February rolls around and the reality of failed resolutions is very noticeable as the attendance begins to decline.

You may ask why I talk so much about New Year's resolutions. I do so because they are typical ways in which people start or re-start an exercise program. It's unfortunate this is often the only time many people give thought to exercise. It should be thought about all year long.

I find it interesting to look at the statistics between exercise dropout rates and the failure rate of New Year's resolutions. In both instances half of all people quit within a few months. Is there a correlation? Probably not, but I think the level of commitment that goes with making a New Year's resolution is similar to the commitment many people make when starting an exercise program. It's superficial, just a good intention to do something. Good intentions rarely result in changes that will last.

To make exercise work, you need more than good intentions to start...you need to make a commitment. A study conducted by Elizabeth Miller, a University of Washington doctoral candidate in psychology, and Alan Marlatt, director of the University's Addictive Behaviors Research Center, found that one of the keys to a successful resolution is commitment to making a change. In addition, Miller states, "Resolutions are a process, not a one-time effort, that offer people a chance to create new habits."

> **Of the millions of Americans who make New Year's resolutions, only 40% will succeed on the first attempt.**

Creating a habit, that's what this chapter is about. If you can successfully make exercise a habit, you are on your way to overcoming many of the obstacles that keep you from being inconsistent. When exercise becomes a habit, the setbacks you face are only speed bumps on the road to making exercise a part of your life.

What Kind of Habits Do You Have?

Webster's defines a habit as "the tendency or disposition to act in a certain way, acquired by repetition of such acts." A habit is developed over time.

Oftentimes, a habit is referred to in a negative way. This can be a habit such as drinking, smoking, or eating the wrong things. Obviously these are habits that can have a negative impact. It's unfortunate, but sometimes we don't realize we are doing these things. We've repeated the action so many times that the behavior has become second nature. Because of this, a habit can be a very powerful thing. And if the habit is a bad one, it can lead to problems.

A habit, as we know, can also be a very good thing. Exercising, brushing your teeth or wearing your seat belt are examples of good habits. In his book *Success is a Choice*, Rick Pitino, former head coach of the Kentucky Wildcats basketball team, talks about how habits develop consistency. But this consistency can work in our favor or against us. It's obvious that the development of consistency with a good habit is positive. However, consistency with a bad habit can result in failure.

If you are involved with a habit that you know is not serving you in a positive way, try to replace it with a good habit. A habit is a habit, right? Its been said that it's easier to eliminate a bad habit if you can immediately replace it with something else, a new habit. Hopefully, then, this new habit will have a positive impact on your life.

What better a habit to start than exercise? Think back to the story at the beginning of the chapter. Maybe the same thing happened to you. Your great intentions to start and stick with an exercise program failed.

Don't be discouraged if this has happened to you. You are not alone. It's amazing how many people give up exercise after only a couple of months. I've seen it over and over. In fact, close to 50% of people drop out of their exercise program in the first 90 days.

Those who give up on exercise after only a short period of time, do so because they haven't fully formed a habit. Remember, habits develop consistency and consistency leads to success. If your New Year's resolution to start an exercise program and lose weight failed, don't worry, at least you took action by trying. Don't look at it as personal weakness that caused you to fail, but rather the inability to develop exercise into a habit.

> **Those who give up on exercise after only a short period of time do so because they haven't fully formed a habit.**

James O. Prochaska, author of over 100 publications, including three books, and internationally recognized for his work as a developer of the stage model of behavior change, says, "People who take action and fail are twice as likely to succeed as people who don't take action at all."

So whether you're a newbie to exercise or you've failed numerous times, let's look at how you can change your life by making exercise a habit.

How to Make Exercise a Habit

For every psychologist out there you will get a different answer on how to adopt a new habit. I've taken the time to look at number of philosophies from the research and taken some of the ideas that will work best when trying to make exercise a habit. So let's look at five steps you can take to make exercise a new habit.

1. You must make a commitment

Before you do anything else, you must commit to the act. In this case it's the act of beginning an exercise program. Tell yourself you are going to do it! Better yet, tell your friends, family members or coworkers you are going to do it. Making a public commitment to begin exercising will make you feel more accountable for your actions. When you tell someone you are going to do something, you are more likely to follow up with it.

Another key to commitment is the language you choose. You need to change from "I want to exercise" or "I think I will exercise" to "I am going to exercise." This is a more positive statement. Too many people are stuck in the "I am thinking about exercise" stage. Don't think, just act!

A great way to act is to pencil in a start date in your day planner or on your calendar and stick to it. You must have a concrete time frame and it must be written down. This shouldn't be the date when you start thinking about where you will exercise. Have it figured out beforehand so you are ready to actually "get physical." Remember, a same time—same place format works very well.

2. Identify the obstacles and overcome!

There will always be something that will get in the way of your new habit. Obstacles may come in the form of an illness, loss of job or relationship problems. Heck, this whole book is about the obstacles you face. There are lots of them and I can almost guarantee something will stand in the way of your progress. No one is immune to adversity.

When adversity strikes you can choose to handle it in a positive or a negative way. If you choose to handle it negatively, then you are setting yourself up for failure. Is that what you want? Of course not! Nobody wants to fail. If you want to be successful, learn to handle adversity in a positive way. Each chapter of this book will serve as a guide to helping you overcome the obstacles that hinder you. Even if you see a chapter that doesn't pertain to you, read it anyway because it may be an issue later on.

We would all like to think there is nothing that can get in the way of making our exercise program work once we get started. Don't be so foolish as to think this is a true statement. Go into your exercise program knowing that something will stifle your progress at some point. Is this being too negative right from the start? I don't think so. It's being realistic. When you are prepared for something, you are better able to overcome it rather than be shocked by it.

You need to accept adversity as a part of life. In his *New York Times* bestselling book, *Body For Life*, Bill Phillips says, "Our character will never be fully tested until things are not going our way. Those who have the courage to succeed in spite of adversity become an inspiration. They contribute value to the lives of others. They make a difference."

When you consistently overcome adversity during the stages of your exercise program, you will become a stronger person, both mentally and physically. This strength will empower you to handle other difficulties you face with exercise and in life.

3. Self-monitoring

It's important to find a way to measure how well you are keeping your commitment. This will help you see the progress you are making.

For example, each time you exercise, record what you do on paper. There are many styles of workout logs to choose from. At the very least, write down in your calendar or daily planner that you exercised on a given day. Doing this will help you see that you are succeeding with your new habit. Later in this book I'll again discuss self-monitoring and you'll see how important it is when boredom and lack of motivation become a barrier to exercise.

When you see that you've succeeded, reward yourself for a job well done. This type of feedback will help reinforce the positive behavior. I consistently preach this to my clients. It really helps.

The reward can come in many different ways. It can be massage therapy, a night out on the town, or buying that something you've always wanted. If you plan to reward yourself for a particular accomplishment, make sure you do it. And do it without regret!

4. You must have perseverance

Calvin Coolidge once said, "Your ability to face setbacks and disappointment without giving up will be the measure of your ability to succeed." How true is this? I guarantee you will face setbacks as you progress through your exercise program. There will be days when you have to miss a workout, maybe even a week or two where you go without exercising. This isn't the end of the world. Just don't give up!

> "Your ability to face setbacks and disappointment without giving up will be the measure of your ability to succeed."
> ~ Calvin Coolidge

For all of you who are worried about taking a few days off and losing what you've gained, you can breathe a sigh of relief. Studies have shown that muscle strength can be maintained with an occasional lapse of as much as 10 to 14 days.

Kicking yourself with comments like, "Here I go again, another missed workout" will get you nowhere. This happens often during the early part of January. People like to make resolutions to begin an exercise program. For the first few days or even a week they do well and stick to it. However, the next week comes along and things get busy, so a workout or two is missed. Feeling bad, they slap their heads and get upset. This leads to a feeling of failure and eventually, if enough workouts are skipped, the end of their desire to work out.

Fact vs. Fiction

Fiction: If you don't weight train for a week you'll lose muscle.

Fact: It takes nearly four weeks without weight training for muscle to atrophy.

Instead of getting frustrated, just pick yourself up and get started again. Don't worry about it. You waste more energy getting upset with yourself than it takes to work out.

Being successful with creating a new habit like exercise has a lot to do with perseverance. Those that succeed are the ones that overcome the little setbacks and press on. Some habits can be formed in a few hours while others may take months. Exercise is one of those habits that takes a little longer. You have to be willing to persevere.

I devote a majority of the final chapter in this book to the importance of perseverance when trying to make exercise a habit.

5. Get social support

People with social support often accomplish more than those who do not. With exercise it's no exception. In fact, studies have shown that you are more likely to succeed with exercise if you have some type of social support.

Social support can come in the form of friends, family members or coworkers. These people can provide support and encouragement during times when you just don't feel like working out.

I've had people at the health club actually call their workout partner if they didn't show up. Because of the phone call that person actually got off the couch

Training Tip

Find a workout partner with similar goals and enthusiasm.

and made their way down to the club and got their workout in for the day. When you know that someone is waiting for you, whether it's at a health club or wherever you choose to work out, you're more likely to be there. Time and time again people tell me that having a workout partner is crucial to their consistency and eventual success.

In my own experience I can testify to this. If I know my partner is waiting for me, I'm not going to let him down. But probably more important is the level of intensity I achieve when I'm with my partner. I can name many times when I would simply go through the motions of lifting weights and not exert a whole lot of effort when I'm alone. It's a different story when my partner is at my side encouraging me to work harder.

The author of Ecclesiastes sums this up well by saying, "Two are better than one, because they have a good return for their work. If one falls down, his friend can help him up. But pity the man who falls and has no one to help him up!"

Self-Control: A Limiting Factor to Your Success?

Self-control refers to the power you have over your thoughts, emotions and behaviors. You use self-control when you initiate or inhibit behavior. This can be behavior such as starting an exercise program. Self-control can determine your likelihood of success. Here's why.

Some psychologists believe that self-control is a limited resource. What they are saying is that every person has only a certain amount of self-control to use each day. Once it's used up, you might as well go to bed or you can forget resisting that chocolate chip cookie dough ice cream in the freezer.

Here is an example. Studies have shown that people who exercise in the morning are more likely to succeed. They succeed, in part, because they haven't had to use up any self-control. This fresh supply of self-control gives them the energy to resist the temptation to skip the workout. The same has been shown for dieters. Bingeing will often occur in the evening hours because much of the dieter's self-control has been used up during the course of the day.

> **Self-control can determine your likelihood of success.**

How many times after a long day at work filled with decisions and deadlines do you just want to plop down on the couch and do whatever comes easy?

Your level of self-control can be depleted throughout the course of a day by the decisions you make. Stress can also do its part of robbing you of your self-control. If you are one of the lucky people out there who have a stress-free life, good for you. As for the rest of us, figure on stress stealing some of your self-control.

Barbara Brehm, Ed.D., professor of exercise and sports studies at Smith College, Northampton, Mass., says, "Coping with stress can leave you emotionally exhausted, and without the energy to get to your workout...stress is the most common reason people slip up in their attempts to overcome addictions or change other habits." These feelings can drain your energy, making it difficult to create a new habit like exercise.

You need to realize that self-control can be a limiting factor to your success with exercise. Reducing the need to use self-control can be of great value. Here is how you can do it.

1. Exercise early in the morning.

2. Know that exercise goes a long way in reducing your stress level.

3. Exercise with a friend—less self-control is needed when you have the encouragement and support of others.

4.   Realize that exercise is hard work—don't kid yourself by saying it's easy. This only puts a drain on your supply of self-control.

Don't Wait...Begin Now!

Trying to make exercise a habit in your life may not be all that easy. Let's be truthful, there are many other habits you form with greater ease. They can be good or bad. The choice is yours.

Following the steps I've outlined for you will not guarantee success. You have to get rid of the excuses and focus on making exercise a habit. Being able to focus on what you want to accomplish is a key ingredient to becoming successful.

Thomas Carlyle said, "The weakest living creature, by concentrating his powers on a single object, can accomplish something; whereas the strongest, by dispersing his over many, may fail to accomplish anything."

Concentrate on making exercise a new habit for you. Put your focus into making it happen. Do this by following the steps I discussed.

1.   Commit yourself.

2.   Set your date to begin and stick to it.

3.   Monitor your progress daily.

4.   Persevere!

5.   Get social support.

You are responsible for making these things happen. No one else can do it for you. Change is not easy, yet it is possible. You just need to go for it!

The "Force Field" of Exercise

I feel that the ability to make exercise a habit is an integral part in helping you overcome many of the barriers that keep you from exercising.

As a child I would have to say my all-time favorite movie was *Star Wars*. I must have seen that movie a dozen times. At the time any movie or television program that had something to do with space was at the top of my list.

One of the features of these movies I thought was just the coolest was the "force field." It was the invisible shield around a space station that deflected anything that tried to attack it. You may have seen this more recently in the movie *Independence Day*, starring Will Smith. If you recall, the United States sent up a bunch of fighter jets to fire missiles into the alien mega-ship. Their shots failed because they were deflected by a force field surrounding the spaceship.

Once you've made exercise a habit it's like having an invisible "force field" around you. Problems that at one time may have caused you to fail no longer have an effect. It seems like you're better able to resist adversities that come your way. This is true because you've been able to develop a tremendous commitment to it. A commitment that takes a lot more than a little adversity to break.

A Habit That Could Save Your Life

I want to conclude this chapter with a story I heard from a speaker at a recent club industry conference I attended. It's a true story that really hit home when I heard it. The story is about the experience a membership salesperson at a health club had with a potential new member.

It was an early October day. The leaves on the trees were already showing dazzling rays of crimson and orange. The temperature in the morning was a chilling 37 degrees with just an occasional peek of sunshine to warm the crisp air. It was the beginning of another day where I looked forward to helping people achieve success and happiness in their life through exercise.

On this day, however, it was a little different. I only had one scheduled appointment with an individual who had kept putting it off for weeks. I looked forward to finally meeting him. He arrived just a few minutes late, hesitating to walk through the doors. After speaking with the gentleman about his health for what seemed like only a few short minutes, I learned how much he needed to begin exercising and make lifestyle changes in his nutritional habits. His cholesterol and blood pressure levels were elevated to what the American Medical Association considers unsafe, he had a family history of heart disease, and he led a life where exercise was regarded as doing a few chores around the house.

In spite of all this, he couldn't commit himself to purchasing a health club membership and exercising. He knew he needed it, yet didn't choose to make it a priority in his life.

After the gentleman left my office 45 minutes later, I wondered why someone who knew his health and activity level weren't the greatest couldn't find it in himself to make exercise a priority.

Well, I followed up with this individual a number of times without success. He just kept saying, "I don't have time." Finally, I thought I would call him one more time. So I called his home, after a number of rings a lady with a soft, sorrowful voice answered. Upon asking to speak with the client, she said "My husband passed away yesterday from a massive heart attack. His arteries were over 95% blocked."

What a feeling of anguish I felt after the phone call, knowing I had had the opportunity to make a difference in the life of this individual.

Even more depressing was the fact that he never made the commitment to "get started." He never made it a priority in his life. He didn't make it a habit and as a result he lost his life.

A Change for the Good

If you want to change your life you, not anyone else, have to take responsibility for your own change. If you've never exercised before, trying to make it a habit will require some change. Henry David Thoreau once said, "Things do not change; we change." Making exercise a habit shouldn't disrupt your life, although it may mean giving something up or rearranging a few priorities.

In his book *Awaken the Giant Within*, Anthony Robbins says this about creating long-term change: "First we must believe that **something must change**...secondly, we must believe that **I must change it**...and third, we have to believe that **I can change it**."

Starting a new exercise program doesn't mean you have to change your life, but your life will be positively changed by it.

CHAPTER 6

I Don't Have Time to Exercise

It Isn't About Time...It's About Priorities!

*"Know the true value of time; snatch, seize, and enjoy
every moment of it. No idleness, no laziness, no pro-
crastination: never put off till tomorrow what you can
do today."*

~ Lord Chesterfield

In all my years working in the fitness industry I have never heard an excuse used more often than, "I don't have time to exercise." Saying that to a person who has given numerous speeches on "Finding Time to Exercise" (that being me) often falls upon deaf ears. Many times I feel like bombarding them with a barrage of questions about their daily routine.

We each have the same number of hours in a day. It's up to you how to spend them.

Did you know that in America today the average person watches approximately 24 to 30 hours of television a week? Wow! You're probably thinking, "That's not me, no way!"

Here is another example of a very popular activity that uses your time. Do you have access to the Internet in your home? A study by Arbitron, a media research firm specializing in music, trends and branding, found that the average person who has broadband (high speed) Internet spends 134 minutes per day online. That is over two hours a day!

If you are one of those people who have used the excuse of not having enough time to exercise, you are not alone. Lack of time is one of the most commonly cited reasons that people either don't start an exercise program or fail to stick with it. Even people with the greatest intentions find themselves being pulled in directions that demand their time. More often than not, exercise is the one thing that gets pushed aside.

How Much Time Do You Have?

I want you to take a few minutes and try the following exercise. It's simple; all you have to do is answer three questions. It will shed some light on the amount of time you have available during the course of a week.

Question A—How many hours are there in one week?

Question B—How many hours do you work each day, on average? Now multiply this by 5.

Question C—How many hours do you sleep each night, on average? Multiply this by 7.

Once you've answered these questions, I'm going to ask you to do a little more math. Don't get worried if math wasn't your thing in school. I want you to plug your answers into the following formula.

Question A - (Question B + Question C)

Let me help you out. I will use myself as an example and insert my answers into the formula. My answers are as follows.

Question A = 168 hours (if you haven't guessed, this will be the same for everyone!)

Question B = 45 hours

Question C = 56 hours

$$168 - (45 + 56) = 67$$

The number "67" represents the amount of free hours I have each week to go about my daily activities outside of work and sleep. That's over 9 hours a day. Your number may be higher or lower. If you think about it, that's a lot of free time you could put toward something meaningful in your life...like exercise.

How Do You Spend Your Free Time?

Now, you are probably thinking all those hours aren't "free time." There are many things that fill the hours between work and sleep. Things like eating, taking care of the kids, errands, working around the house, paying bills, organizational meetings, entertainment, and many others. They all take time, making your "free time" hours dwindle quite rapidly.

You need to look at what is reducing your free time and determine if it is a priority or not. If you say you don't have time for something, it's probably not that you don't have time, it's that you don't make it a priority. We all find time for the things we want to do.

An effective exercise program will take you only three hours a week provided it's done correctly. This represents only 4.4% of the time you have available each week if your sleep and work schedule is similar to mine. That's it! Just think of the benefits you can receive by using less than 5% of your time on a worthy cause. Fitness magazines and health sections of the newspaper are overflowing with reasons why you should exercise. So, what are you waiting for? Make exercise a priority.

> **We all find time for the things we want to do.**

Why Make Exercise a Priority?

How many times have you woken up in the morning and not even given a thought to the fact that you are healthy? Just think about it. Do you regularly jump out of bed and say, "Oh good, I can breathe today!" or "Thank goodness, I can get out of bed this morning." Well, maybe some mornings getting out of bed can be a challenge for all of us. My point is that we often take our health for granted. Another day passes and we go about our usual routine without really thinking what it would be like if we had an illness preventing us from doing the things we like to do.

I know you have heard about the benefits of exercise over and over. Like how it can prevent many of the most common causes of premature death and disability like cardiovascular disease, type II diabetes, obesity, hypertension and some types of cancer.

Recently I came across a study that stated that people who exercise are less likely to die at an early age than sedentary people. The study observed large groups of men and women over a 15-year period to determine the health outcomes of active compared to sedentary people. It found that sedentary men were three times as likely to have died over a 15-year period than those who exercised regularly. Sedentary women were four times as likely to die over the same period as their more active counterparts.

Earlier in this book I mentioned how cancer is the second leading cause of death in the United States. Undoubtedly you know someone or have a loved one that has had cancer in their life. As I write this book there is no cure for cancer, but there is a way to help protect yourself from it. That way is by incorporating exercise in your life.

In 2002, the American Cancer Society estimated that the most commonly occurring cancers in men were prostate, lung and colon cancer, while breast, lung and colon cancer were most prevalent in women.

A study by the Harvard School of Public Health, Harvard Medical School and Brigham and Women's Hospital examined whether physical activity plays a role in the prevention of cancer. The study found that physically active men and women have a 30 to 40% reduction in the risk of developing colon cancer, compared to inactive persons. In regard to breast cancer, evidence shows that physically active women have about a 20 to 30% reduction in risk.

I find it interesting that the most common cancers to inflict us are the very ones that may be prevented by regular exercise.

I can write a list of reasons citing why you should exercise that would encompass several pages of this book; however, I won't because chances are you're well aware of them already. In fact, I have a poster I received through one of my trade journals that lists 100 reasons why you should exercise.

Thinking Practically

Let's take a more practical look at why you may consider making exercise a priority in your life.

1. Stress relief

Take, for example, stress. We all have it. If you don't then you must live in a box or don't come in contact with the world around you. Even if you lived in isolation, you would probably find a way to get stressed out.

Stress can do a lot of damage in our lives. It can lead to feelings of depression that reduce your motivation levels. If you have a job requiring you to meet weekly or monthly goals, stress can greatly hinder your potential to achieve them. In fact, stress-related illnesses cost U.S. businesses nearly 500 million employee workdays each year.

> **"If you don't have health, it's difficult to operate in a high-stress environment."**
> **~ Dr. Bob Boni**

What if you are hoping to get a promotion, yet you are faced with a difficult situation? All of a sudden your stress level skyrockets. Your ability to perform effectively may be compromised.

Stress can also lead to emotional weakness. For example, say you just got over an addiction such as smoking, drinking or overeating. Many times people will fall back on that type of addiction in order to deal with the stress.

Guess what? Exercise can reduce feelings of stress and anxiety. It can take your mind off the problems you're faced with. Your body is better able to respond to stress when you are physically active.

Dr. Michael H. Sacks says this about exercise and stress, "Exercise can be a powerful method of relaxation, and it can help people deal effectively with the stress of daily life. In various studies, researchers have found that exercise can decrease anxiety and depression, improve an individual's self-image, and buffer people from the effects of stress...Exercise increases blood flow to the brain, releasing hormones and stimulating the nervous system...".

You don't have to let stress destroy the quality of your life. Regular exercise acts as a buffer against stress and helps protect the body against its consequences.

2. Better quality time

If you have children you know how active they can be. Sometimes I wish I had the ability to bottle up their energy and use it for myself. Just think of all the extra work that could be accomplished if this were possible. Although exercise may not bring back that childlike energy, it can do wonders to boost your current energy levels.

I often ask new members of my health club, after a month or so, what they feel has been the biggest change in their life since starting an exercise program. Without question, the most common response is that they have more energy. This answer comes after only a few weeks of exercise.

Having more energy allows you to do more on a daily basis, therefore making you more productive. On the same note, how many times have you come home from work and had your kids tugging at your pants saying, "Let's play"? After a long day at work you just don't have the energy to do it. But, because you haven't seen them all day you agree to play for a while. Despite the fact that you agree to play with them, your heart just isn't into it. Don't fool yourself into thinking they can't see this.

Patrick Morley, in his book *Seven Seasons of a Man's Life*, talks about the value of spending time with your family. He says that, "Many dads today suffer from the Weekend Day Syndrome. They slave away at their work so hard Monday through Friday that they rarely see their kids except on weekends. They become two-day-a-week dads...Time is everything to a relationship, whether with your wife or kids."

Though in this passage Morley refers only to dads, this can be equally true for working moms.

The results of a lack of energy after only a normal workday can be similar to what Morley discusses about those who work extra-long hours. The point is that proper attention is not given to your family.

Family time, especially time spent with your kids, needs to be enjoyed and cherished. Those of you who have grown children

> "Time is everything to a relationship."
> ~ Patrick Morley

know how fast they grow up. Wouldn't you like to have the energy and enthusiasm to play with them day after day? What parent wouldn't? Or, how important is it to have the energy to engage in lively conversation with your spouse when they need to talk?

The fact is our lives are so busy we often lack the energy needed to do all the things we'd like. We need to determine the priorities in our lives and put them first. Making exercise a priority will increase your energy level so you have the energy necessary for quality time with an even higher priority in your life...your children or spouse.

3. Being successful

Without a doubt most people reading this book want to be successful. Success can come in the form of good health, wealth, a great family life, a particular career or in many other ways. Success, however, comes with a price. You first must be able to define what it means to be successful. Once you've done this you need to work hard to achieve it. The hard work you dedicate toward it may take months or, most likely, years to accomplish. Finally, when you think you've come to the point of being successful, you realize it was just the start. Everyone has heard the saying—success is a journey, not a destination. We'll discuss this more in the final chapter.

The truth is that if you aren't healthy, you won't be able to work with the enthusiasm and tenacity it takes to become successful.

Think of a time when you were not feeling well, maybe you had the flu. Despite this you still had some work that needed to be done at the office. How productive were you? My guess is you weren't productive at all. It's difficult to get motivated when you are not feeling well.

Pat Croce began his career as a local physical therapist, later becoming the owner of the Philadelphia 76ers professional basketball team. He took them from a team that won only 22 games in his first season to the NBA finals in 2001. This was the team's first visit to the finals since 1982-83 season. What a success Pat Croce had become.

With a deeply rooted background in fitness, Pat has this to say about the relationship between success and exercise:

"I truly believe one of the foundations of my success is having a fit body, therefore a fit mind. The mind and body are one, so that a fit body will bring a fit mind. It's difficult to feel great if you're injured and in pain. You can't feel great if you're tired. If your body is in shape through physical fitness, sports or outdoor activities, you'll have that much more energy with which to follow your dream; more energy to work harder, play harder, study longer and fulfill your goals."

Exercise won't make you immune to becoming sick; however, it can decrease the frequency and severity of illness. Being healthy will allow you to accomplish more and create an environment for success.

> "I truly believe one of the foundations of my success is having a fit body, therefore a fit mind."
> ~ Pat Croce

Why does exercise create such a positive feeling? It's the little hormones called endorphins. They are proteins found in the brain, spinal cord and endocrine glands that act as natural painkillers, mood elevators and tranquilizers, all in one. Endorphins are said to increase mental and physical energy as well as enhance creativity. Furthermore, the same things that produce endorphins also boost your immune system. And guess what? Exercise causes a release of these endorphins.

With all the positive changes that occur because of exercise, you become better equipped to work harder at achieving success in your life. Wouldn't you agree this is a fair tradeoff for dedicating only a few hours a week toward exercise?

Identifying Priorities That Matter

I do a lot of reading in the area of leadership because I feel it is my God-given gift. I have read countless books in this area. Without a doubt my favorite author is John Maxwell. He is an amazing writer and really knows how to get his point across. In his book *Leadership 101*, John says that "The discipline to prioritize and the ability to work toward a stated goal are essential to a leader's success."

Now, I know we are not talking about leadership in this book, but the principle remains the same—you must look at exercise as a priority in your life if you want to be successful.

Maybe you need to think about it a different way. Rather than just thinking *exercise* should be a priority, look at it as your *health* being a priority. As I mentioned before, many people in society today take their health for granted. People are so accustomed to waking up in the morning and not thinking twice about the breath of air they just took. I am guilty of it myself. It's not until you become sick or injured that you realize how lucky you are to be healthy.

You've probably heard of people who you thought were healthy die unexpectedly from a heart attack. It's not until later you find out their death wasn't unexpected at all. Silently over the years their eating habits or lack of consistent exercise contributed to the build-up of plaque in their arteries, ultimately leading to the attack.

> "Things which matter most must never be at the mercy of things which matter least."
> ~ Goethe

You don't have to feel sick to be sick. Many diseases develop without our knowledge. Don't let yourself go down without out a fight. Make time for the improvement of your health.

German poet and novelist Johann Wolfgang von Goethe gives all of us a concept to consider when he says, "Things which matter most must never be at the mercy of things which matter least."

What are the things that matter most in your life? What are your priorities? Your family and friends, your spiritual life, maybe it is your career or your health? The choice is yours.

Most adults have between six and twelve priorities. With that many priorities, how do you know what to put first? Making your health a priority will make all the other things you cherish more enjoyable and lasting.

How to Put the
Important Things First

1. The Pareto principle

The Pareto principle, originally stated by Italian economist Vilfredo Pareto, says that 80% of the reward comes from 20% of your effort IF you put all your effort into that top 20%.

A good example of this principle in my line of work is that 20% of health club members are responsible for 80% of the product sales.

What you need to do is figure out the 20% of activities in your life that will give you 80% of the results. But, before you do this you need to know what type of results you are after. Is it career advancement, becoming wealthy, a great family life, a closer walk with the Lord or a healthy life?

Everybody will have a different answer. I can tell you one answer that may help in many of these areas...that is exercise. Earlier in this chapter we looked at how it contributes to stress relief, increased energy and the potential to becoming successful. Without your health many of these things aren't possible. What is your top 20%?

2. Is It urgent or important?

It is essential that you identify those activities in your life that are urgent and those that are important. Urgent means that it has to be dealt with now. These things insist that we take action. An example would be the phone ringing. Most people would not just let it ring—they would answer it. Pressing problems at work would be another example. Urgent matters demand our time; however, they are often not important.

Important matters, on the other hand, generally consist of things that have value to us. They have to do with results. These are the activities that should have a high priority in our lives; they build into our goals and values. Important matters are activities such as planning, relationship building and dare I say...exercise?

In his book *The Seven Habits of Highly Effective People*, Stephen Covey talks about these two types of activities in what he calls the time management matrix. Covey places them in quadrants. Quadrant I are urgent and important activities. Quadrant II consists of things that are important but not urgent. Quadrant III are activities that are urgent but not important. Quadrant IV are the activities that are not important and not urgent. Covey goes on to say that the activities in quadrant II are most valuable to us. It deals with the things that are not urgent, but important. Things like building relationships, long-range planning, preventative maintenance, and even Stephen Covey places exercise in this category. He says the quadrant II activities are things we know we need to do, but rarely get to because we get sidetracked with things that are urgent and not important.

Take time to make a list of your day-to-day activities and separate the urgent from the important ones. Give time to the activities that are important but not urgent. They are the ones that make a positive impact in your life. Robert J. McKain once said, "The reason most major goals are not achieved is that we spend our time doing second things first." Do you?

3. Write your priorities down on paper

This is as simple as it seems. Write down on paper the things you see as your highest priorities. After you've done this place it in a spot where you will see it every day. This spot can be on your bathroom mirror, the dashboard of your car or on your refrigerator. You need to be reminded of your priorities on a regular basis or else you will get distracted by the "urgent" things that don't build into your goals or values.

4. Align your priorities with your behavior

Once you've identified your highest priorities, you need to incorporate them into your lifestyle. They need to become part of your everyday behavior pattern. With time and consistency they will soon become habitual. The advantage of this is the little distractions that get in your way, things that have sidetracked you

> "Until you learn to prioritize, you will be constantly distracted and interrupted by trivialities."
> ~ Vince Lombardi, Jr.

in the past, will now become avoidable. Aligning your priorities with your behavior will give you time for the things that are important in life. Past excuses like "I don't have time to exercise" will not be a part of your vocabulary because you know it's something that leads to positive changes in your life.

Know What's Important and Act on It

It is my hope that after reading the four steps I've outlined about identifying your priorities, you'll be able to uncover the activities that are important to you and learn how to make them part of your daily routine.

Once you've written down your list of priorities, take time to think and place each of them in order of importance.

More often than not, people have too many priorities and it can be paralyzing. You know, the "to-do" lists that require more

> "Anything that is excellent or praiseworthy stands moment-by-moment on the cutting edge and must be constantly fought for."
> ~ H. Ross Perot

hours to accomplish than we have in a day. Earlier I told you that most adults have six to 12 priorities. Don't worry if you are one of them. Sit down, look at your list of priorities, reflect on them and determine which ones mean the most to you.

I need to warn you, however. Just when you think you are set and living your priorities in the right order, they change. Yes, that's right. Priorities will change depending on what stage of life you're in. Getting married, raising children or moving to a different location all play a role. H. Ross Perot said, "Anything that is excellent or praiseworthy stands moment-by-moment on the cutting edge and must be constantly fought for." If change occurs, don't worry about it. Just make changes to your list based on your life stage. Plan on doing this each year. Over time you will find that some of the priorities on your list will always remain the same. Those may be family, friends, spirituality, and hopefully exercise.

Make Room for Your Priorities

The things in your life you consider priorities are going to take a significant amount of time. They should if they are priorities. If you find yourself constantly having more to do than time to do it in, then you need to reprioritize or develop some good time management skills. Having good time management skills will allow you to make the best use of your time. Hopefully you can dedicate some of this time to exercise. Let's look at ways you can do this.

1. Prioritize

I know we talked about this already, but it's crucial when trying to manage your time. You have to know what comes first in your life. If you don't then you will spend most of your time doing second things first. Remember the 80/20 rule: 80% of the reward comes from 20% of the effort.

2. Plan and organize

I'm sure you've heard this quote, "If you fail to plan, you're planning to fail." It has lots of truth to it. Just think of an average day at work. You go to work, sit down at your desk and look at all the papers, memos and other distracting information all strewn about. You sit there for a half hour looking things over, rearranging the piles and wasting

> **If you fail to plan, you are planning to fail.**

time just trying to get things organized. Is this a familiar scene? I know I am guilty of it on occasion. This is where good planning and organization comes in handy. Taking the time to think and plan is time well spent. You will eliminate the wasted time because you know in advance what you need to do. This allows you to immediately start on what is important.

3. Make a to-do list

There are many ways you can go about utilizing a to-do list. Some people will end their day by creating a to-do list for the next day, while others will make it first thing in the morning. There also are people who will keep a running list of weekly things to do. As the week goes on they add to it as necessary. By the end of the week everything should be crossed off. Or, some will incorporate a to-do list in their weekly planner. They'll get as specific as scheduling things at a certain time of the day. You need to find what works best for you. Try different methods; if one fails try something else.

Now, having a to-do list or scheduling activities in a planner are not just for those who work outside the home. The stay-at-home mom or dad can also be a better manager of their time by doing the same thing. Granted, your "things to do" will be quite different; however, the principle is the same.

Having a to-do list is a great method for accomplishing tasks in a timely manner. Since I began doing this I've found that I am much more effective and can make better use of my time.

4. Learn to say "no"

This is a hard one for most people, including myself. You don't want to disappoint somebody, but yet you already have too much on your plate. We have to remember that we cannot please everyone. Doing so is failure to define what is important to you. Saying no isn't necessarily a selfish thing; you need to draw the line between what is considered helping people and being used.

Here are a few ways you can say "no" without hurting anyone's feelings.

- Decide what you need to get accomplished in a given day or week and say no to whatever interferes.

- Think about how you say no. It's usually the tone in your voice or your body language that alienates someone, not the fact that you told them no. Say to them, "Thank your for the opportunity (or invitation); unfortunately, it is not a good time for me."

- Make it clear to people, when you are saying no, that it doesn't mean you will never help them. Be graceful and open to the opportunity to help at a different time. This will most always end in a positive experience.

Saying no is tough to do and I'll be the first to admit it. However, the more you do it the easier it gets. Do it in a graceful and compassionate way and you will not only have a positive experience, but you will create more time to spend exercising.

5. Leave the little stuff

Over the course of a day there are many little things we find ourselves involved with. These things end up wasting valuable time. They can be classified as urgent and not important. They only have short-term implications. We need to focus on the things that are important and accomplish them first. Highlight them on your to do list and give them priority in your day.

Set aside a block of time during your day to accomplish the little things and focus on getting them done quickly. Do this only after the important tasks are complete.

6. Be flexible

You have to allow time for interruptions, distractions and emergencies. Expect the unexpected. I get this all the time working at a health club. I'll be sitting in my office working on a project and all of a sudden in pops a client. "Hey Tim, can you give me a spot?" or "I'm not sure how I should be doing this exercise, can you give me a hand?" This happens all the time. To be truthful, I don't mind it. After all, my job is to help people, however difficult it becomes to complete my office work.

I'm sure a similar situation like this has happened to you whether you are at work or in the home. It's important that we plan our day knowing that we will be interrupted. Time management experts say that you should plan to use only 50% of your time. Therefore, when you get distracted, you will still have time to accomplish the important things.

If Not Now, When?

Many busy people manage to make time for exercise. In her book *Healthy, Wealthy and Wise*, Krs Edstrom interviewed some of the top CEOs in the country from companies such as GTE, Boeing, Coca-Cola, General Foods and J.C. Penney. One common denominator among these CEOs was that they made time to exercise. It was one of their important tasks. Now, you can imagine the busyness of their daily schedule, yet they make time to exercise. Why? Because more than 93% of them say their success can be attributed to being healthy.

Randy Barron, former president of Southwestern Bell Company, says, "You should make taking care of your body a priority. One hour out of twenty-four isn't that much—my contribution to this corporation depends on my good physical shape." Even if you dedicate one hour only three times a week, you will see positive changes in your body.

> ## Fitness Fact
>
> **97% of Americans place maintaining good physical health among their top personal priorities.**

Many people say they are too busy to exercise. When in the future will you be less busy? More than likely things will get busier before they slow down. We are a society that spreads ourselves too thin. If you wait to begin exercising, you may be waiting forever.

Why wait? You need to think about your future and your long-term goals. Your health will play an integral role toward achieving these goals. People who don't make exercise a priority are more likely to find themselves sick, depressed, or stressed out. How productive can you be in this condition? Suddenly the priorities that were once first in your life become secondary to getting healthy again. Author John Lubbock couldn't have put it better when he said, "In cultivating the mind we must not neglect the body. Those who do not have time for exercise will have to find time for illness."

Take the couple extra hours a week to become involved with exercise. It will keep you healthier, allowing you to enjoy all the great things life has to offer. Use your time wisely.

CHAPTER 7

I'm Not Motivated to Exercise

How to Map Your Way
to Becoming Motivated

*"The most important thing about motivation is goal
setting. You should always have a goal."*
~ Francie Larrieu Smith

All right, let's get real here. How do people get motivated to work out? We're talking sweat, burning muscles, post-workout soreness and heavy breathing to name a few of the more unpleasant side effects of exercise. This not so wonderful description is the reason why very few people can truly say they are motivated to exercise. Sure, there are a few individuals out there that thrive on feeling the pain and subject themselves to it day after day and week after week. But what about the majority of people? Which category do you fall in?

When it comes to not exercising on a regular basis, I see two types of people. The first are those who aren't motivated and don't feel the need to get involved. This makes up about one fifth of the population. These are the people who are completely sedentary. They have absolutely no desire to exercise now or anytime in the future. They don't see it as important and probably never will.

The second type are those who have made the effort to start an exercise program, but couldn't keep it going. They quit due to lack of results, boredom or lack of interest or enjoyment. According to John McCarthy of the International Health, Racquet & Sportsclub Association, 50% of people who start an exercise program at a health club quit within six months of joining. Of the 50% who quit, 70% of them do so because they lose motivation.

Do you fall into one of these categories? If you do, don't feel bad—you are in the majority. However, in this case you don't want to be a part of the majority. Being a part of it isn't going to improve the quality of your life. You need to consider your position and be openminded to what I am about to tell you so that motivation, or lack thereof, is no longer a barrier to exercise for you.

How Are You Motivated?

The dictionary defines motivation as the act or process of providing an incentive to stimulate action. When you think back to my opening comments about how exercise makes you sweat and causes your muscles to be sore, how can this be an incentive to stimulate action?

For many years our society has studied motivation. It's a crucial element to becoming successful. Business owners want to know what motivates their employees. Likewise, teachers want to know how they can motivate their students to learn. In the same way, personal trainers look for ways to motivate their clients so they keep exercising.

Motivation is often broken down into two categories: external and internal motivation. External motivation is when a person is motivated for reasons like social approval, material rewards or status. For example, people may be motivated by the possibility of becoming popular, a raise in pay, a bonus, trophies or a promotion.

On the other hand, you have those who are motivated by internal reasons such as personal pride, sheer joy for what they are doing, a strong work ethic or the personal mastery involved with the experience.

Over the years I've spent working in health clubs and counseling people, I've found that many people are externally motivated usually in the form of vanity. People want to look good for their wedding or vacation. That social approval is important to them, in many cases more important than what's happening inside their bodies. By this I mean the positive physiological effects exercise can have on your health. Unfortunately, these external motivators are ones that don't often endure. They may work in the short term and fade as time goes on. This explains why many people give up on exercise so quickly.

I came across something interesting while reading through a chapter in Zig Ziglar's book *Over the Top.* If you don't know who Zig Ziglar is you're missing out. He is one of the greatest motivational speakers on the planet!

In a chapter on motivation he talks about how people who attend his seminars have said that listening to his motivational tapes have helped them to lose weight. Some of these people said they've lost as much as 50 pounds. Zig mentions that he "assumed they

> **Being motivated can actually help you lose weight!**

had been inspired to change their eating and exercise habits when actually the body's chemical response to motivation itself was an important factor."

Zig says that the motivational seminar or audiotape activates chemicals in the brain like endorphins, dopamine, and norepinephrine. These chemicals, when released, increase your energy and endurance.

Let's look at how you can increase your motivation for exercise while at the same time activate chemicals in the brain that will enhance other areas of your life.

Lasting Motivation

If you want to make exercise a part of your life, it is imperative that you do it for internal reasons. John Baucom, author of *Baby Steps to Success,* says, "Motivation is an internal source of energy. It's composed of inner desires, urges, energy, and instincts." You have to want to do it. Your inner desires are the most powerful and most often lead to lasting effects.

Lasting success will come from being internally motivated. Richard M. Ryan, professor of psychology at the University of Rochester, says, "To really keep an exercise program going, it needs to be something you are doing because you value the actual activity—you appreciate the exercise for the sake of exercising."

I firmly believe this; however, I need to make a point. For those of you who are trying to get started with exercise, maybe for the first time, you will need more than internal motivation because that is what you lack in the first place. The very reason you're not motivated is because you don't have internal desire to exercise. You're not going to be magically motivated to exercise just because someone tells you that it's important. This is a time where it may be beneficial to use some kind of external motivator to get you going. Let me give you some examples.

External Motivators
to Get You Jump-Started

At my health club we often run what we call retention games. They are games where members are challenged to stay active and use the facility by offering games where prizes can be won.

It's amazing what a small prize such as some coupons for free smoothies or tanning can do to motivate people. Well, it's not just the prizes that do it, but also the fact that their names appear on a bulletin board where other club members see their progress in the game.

We have had a number of these games over the years and it never fails how well they work. People get excited and go to great lengths to make sure they complete the tasks necessary to stay in contention for the prize.

We once had a game called the "Amazing Waist." The idea was brilliant, though I have to admit I can't take the credit for thinking of the game; it was one of my employees. The game was simple. All you had to do was lose at least ¼ pound of body weight each week in order to remain eligible for the final prize—a lifetime membership to the health club. Each week the members who entered would have to be weighed in by a staff person. If the member did not lose at least ¼ pound, they were eliminated. It was as simple as that. We had tons of people sign up for the contest and, finally, after nine months, a winner was crowned. During the time those who entered the contest worked hard and were consistent with their exercise program. It was the combination of external rewards (the big prize, and the recognition from peers) and internal rewards (a sense of pride and achievement) that made the contest so effective.

Another game we often run is one in which the members need to complete a certain amount of time on the cardiovascular and strength training equipment during the course of a week. Each week if they complete the requirements they receive a star on their game sheet. Requirements range from completing 20 minutes of cardiovascular exercise three times a week, taking an aerobic class or utilizing the strength training equipment twice a week. It was amazing to see the effort people put forth just to complete their game sheets. People tell me that they actually went out of their way to exercise so they could stay in the game and qualify for the prize. The prizes I'm talking about were usually nothing grandiose.

Organized competition is another source of external motivation to help you get started or maintain your motivation to exercise. One way is to make it a goal to run in a local 5k race or triathlon. There are very few people who will set their sights on some type of event and not want to do well. If it isn't your thing to compete then you can sign up for a charity walk/run. By signing up you know you'll have to exert some physical effort to complete the course, therefore encouraging you to train for it. In the process you help yourself and others.

One more type of external motivator that has been made popular by Bill Phillips, former owner and CEO of EAS, a supplement company, is the Body For Life Challenge. You may have heard of the contests Bill organizes through his former magazine, *Muscle Media*. The contest is a challenge to see who can transform his or her body and make the greatest change in a 12-week period. Along with the transformation you are required to write an essay titled "Why I Entered the Body For Life Challenge." The contest is judged by a panel of people who subjectively look at photos, measurements, and read your essay. Thousands of people have entered over the years and used the contest to begin lifelong exercise and nutrition habits. They just needed that spark, or in this case the contest, to get motivated. Just a little note: some of the prizes for placing high in the competition were items like Corvettes, Hawaiian vacations, and large amounts of money. Not a bad motivator, huh?

Remember, using an external factor to get motivated is only a short-term solution. Jay Williams, Ph.D., author of the *24 Hour*

Turnaround, reports that "70% of those who make a lifestyle change for external reasons do not stick with it after a short period of time." Real success will only come from exercising for internal reasons. This is something that you will not feel immediately. It has to grow on you. You need to experience success, gratification, and enjoyment in order to truly internalize the feeling that exercise can bring.

The Power of Encouragement

Sometimes it seems impossible to get motivated, regardless of what we are getting motivated for. When this happens you need to surround yourself with caring, positive people who will be an encouragement to you. Everyone we come in contact with has an influence on us. That influence can be good or bad. Be sure to surround yourself with people who will encourage you in a positive way.

I recently read a story about how encouragement can be so powerful. A group of psychologists wanted to look at a person's ability to endure pain. So they took a bucket of ice water and had people stand in it, barefooted, as long as they could. What they found was that the people who were encouraged to "hang in there" a little longer actually did last longer than those who had no encouragement.

Let's take a look at three examples of how you can become motivated to exercise by the encouragement of others.

1. Positive relationships

You probably know a friend or family member who is an avid exerciser and seems to enjoy it. Spend more time with this individual. Allow their zeal for exercise to rub off on you. You'd be amazed at how much

> "When a person feels encouraged, he can face the impossible and overcome incredible adversity."
> ~ John Maxwell

another person can influence your life when it comes to exercise. If you associate with people who despise and have no desire to exercise, then you can bet beginning an exercise program will be very difficult.

Even for me lack of motivation is a problem I face occasionally. Often this lack of motivation isn't in the form of getting started with exercise, but rather being motivated enough to have a quality workout session. There is no doubt in my mind that the people who surround me during my workout (i.e., my training partner and others in the gym) can make or break the workout. I have some partners that are great encouragers, while others just allow me to go through the motions without much encouragement. It's a night and day difference when I evaluate the workout after I'm finished.

Make it a point to surround yourself with people who enjoy exercise and have made it a part of their lives.

2. Find a mentor

Having a mentor offers an incredible opportunity to succeed at something you may think is impossible on your own. A mentor will be your guiding light; they'll get you through the tough times and encourage you when you fail.

> **Make it a point to surround yourself with people who enjoy exercise and have made it a part of their lives.**

Whom should you look for? What qualities does this person need to have? First, find someone whom you get along with. It should be someone you can relate to and not be afraid to express your thoughts and feelings to. Second, this person should be knowledgeable and experienced with exercise. Finally, make sure they have been consistent over a long period of time with their own exercise program. You need a strong person who has proven they can incorporate exercise into his or her life.

Take the time to talk and spend time with this person. Maybe they can become your workout partner, or simply, someone you know you can call when you need encouragement or have questions.

Find someone who fits this description and tell that person you have admired their exercise efforts and would like to learn from and be encouraged by them. They will be flattered and happy to help.

3. Find a group of people to hang with

What I mean by this is to find a group of people who have the same interest in exercising as you. It can be a group of people at your local health club or people who regularly get together and walk or go on bike rides. It's also a good idea that these people have something in common with you and are at similar fitness levels. This makes it easier for you to get along as well as keep up with each other. The whole experience will be more enjoyable if you heed this advice.

Keep in mind, the group doesn't necessarily have to consist of people you exercise with. Take Weight Watchers for example— look how successful that organization has become. Just think, you are surrounded by like-minded people who have taken the steps to make nutrition a lifestyle. The positive and encouraging attitudes in a group are priceless.

Check with your local health club or nutrition store to see if there is some kind of exercise or nutrition focus group in your area. If there is, get involved!

Finding a Vision

Once you've sparked a little motivation to get going on your own or have been encouraged by others, you need to nurture this motivation in order for it to stay alive and well. If you're someone who has already started exercising or has started and failed, what I'm about to say can help you to get motivated again. It all starts with vision...you have to know where you are going.

> "Vision without action is a daydream. Action without vision is a nightmare."
> ~ Japanese proverb

Everything starts with a vision. Some may go as far as calling it a dream. It's your ability to see something you want to achieve that may be just out of reach. An old Japanese proverb says: "Vision without action is a daydream. Action without vision is a nightmare." In order to be successful with your action (starting an exercise program), you need to have a vision.

Ask yourself what you want to accomplish by exercising. Do you want to lose weight? Get stronger? Build endurance? Have more energy? Look and feel good? Compete in an athletic event? The list is endless. If you can't seem to get started with exercise or have failed time and time again, you need to set a clear, concise vision that allows you to look forward to the future. Vince Lombardi, Jr. says, "Vision is a future reality yet to come into existence."

I know many people set what they call "goals," and do so in such a light manner that it really doesn't mean much. Even those who exercise consistently can stray from their efforts when a clear vision of what they are exercising for isn't identified. It's something that you need to make so real that you can see, smell, taste and touch it in your mind.

Let's look at two ways a vision can encourage you to be motivated for exercise.

The Power to Keep You Going

When it comes to exercise, it takes tenacity. No matter who you are or how long you have been exercising, something will come up and you will end up taking a hiatus. What determines whether you will get going again is your vision. If you have a strong vision of where you want to go it will give you the strength to make it through times of personal doubt and feelings of laziness.

So many people quit their exercise program after only six weeks because they lose interest or don't see the results they thought were possible. You need to realize that results don't always come quickly. I know we live in a "now" society; that is, we want everything now and don't want to wait. If you want to see results with exercise, you have to work for them. This is where having a vision is important. If you have a vision that is very clear and real to you then it will become the fuel you need to drive you day after day, week after week and beyond. I truly think that the ability to keep going when the going gets tough is the key to being successful at making exercise a part of your life. A word for this is perseverance. I have an entire chapter dedicated to it at the end of this book.

Another way that vision can be powerful in helping you to exercise is its ability to help you set goals. Bill Phillips, in his bestselling book, *Body For Life*, says, "When you develop a strong future vision, you don't have to force yourself to set goals, your mind just compels you to set them. And every time you accomplish an objective, it's not the end of anything; it's the beginning, the starting point for another stage of an ongoing journey of progress, development, growth, and adventure."

Goal setting is critical for the new exerciser as well as the seasoned veteran. But, in order for goal setting to work you must first have a vision.

Let me ask you this: when you decide to go on a vacation, do you just pack your bags and start driving? No! You first envision where you want to go, and then take the steps necessary to get there.

The same is true with exercise; you need to know where you want to go. Maybe it is to lose a certain amount of weight or to do well in a competition. It can be many different things, but it should be only one thing. This one thing is what will drive you each day. In order for this vision to become reality you need to map out a way to get there. You need to set some goals that will bridge the gap between your current status and the one you envision happening.

Find Motivation Through Goal Setting

What is it that separates someone who is motivated to exercise and one who isn't? The answer is a clear sets of goals. Everybody who is consistently motivated to exercise on a day-to-day basis has one or more sets of goals in mind. In his book, *Success Is a Choice*, Rick Pitino says, "Goals are our day-by-day blueprint that provide achievable targets for incremental improvement." Setting goals will allow you to make your vision an achievable possibility.

Paul Myer once said, "No one ever accomplishes anything of consequence without a goal...goal setting is the strongest human force for self-motivation." What is one of the greatest motivators you can think of? Success! Who isn't motivated when they experience success?

For example, you envision yourself losing 25 pounds and looking fantastic for your upcoming vacation to an island in the Caribbean. At first, this seems like it may be an insurmountable task because you have so much weight to lose and you love to eat pizza. When you look at this task and break it down into smaller more manageable steps (each step being a goal), you are increasing your chances of being successful. Why? Because each time you accomplish a small goal, you experience success and this success creates motivation to continue.

These small goals can be as simple as working out three times a week, cutting back on simple carbohydrates, or adding several minutes to your treadmill walk each week. By accomplishing small goals little by little you are taking a big step to realizing

> "No one ever accomplishes anything of consequence without a goal...goal setting is the strongest human force for self-motivation."
> ~ Paul Myer

your vision of being 25 pounds lighter on the beach in Aruba.

I found a great illustration that describes how succeeding a little at a time can lead to a big accomplishment. The illustration comes from Vince Lombardi, Jr. and John Baucom's book, *Baby Steps to Success*. It goes like this.

Many professional football coaches have had a dream of winning an NFL championship. This resulted in the goal of winning their division. There was an even smaller goal of winning a certain number of games, which was then subdivided into winning several particular games. This resulted from goals of making touchdowns and extra points. That goal was reduced to making a series of first downs and ultimately the necessity of gaining two or three yards on a particular play.

So how does a football team win a championship? They start by first having the simple goal gaining a few yards per play. Success from doing this empowers them to work toward the next goal. The goal of getting a first down. And so on.

Finding motivation to exercise is very similar. You first need to set some achievable goals and then experience success with those goals. This pattern will provide a positive flow of energy and motivation to help you become consistent with exercise. Maybe even something you look forward to! Let's look at how you can set goals that become the stepping-stones to realizing your vision.

Mapping Your Way to Motivation

Vance Havner said, "The vision must be followed by the venture. It is not enough to stare up the steps. We must step up the stairs." Each step you take represents an accomplished goal. Accomplish enough goals and you will soon be at the top. This is what you need to do.

Before you map out the steps that lead to making your vision a reality, you have to know what that vision is. You can't set incremental goals without having vision. So take some time to really think about what it is you want to accomplish. Don't underestimate your ability, but, on the other hand, don't over-estimate it and shoot for something that is unreasonable. Losing 10 pounds in two months is reasonable; losing 30 pounds in six weeks is not. Set yourself up for success.

Defining your goals

This is the most critical step to making the whole thing work. It provides the framework that you will follow. Steven Covey, in his book *First Things First,* talks about how it's important to know the "what, why and how" of the things you want to accomplish. Let's look at this idea and put it into an example that will help you understand its concept.

The "what" asks the question, what is it that I want to accomplish? Or, what end do I have in mind? Using the example from earlier in the chapter, the "what" question would go like this. "I would like to begin an exercise and nutrition program so I can lose 25 pounds before my vacation." What is *your* "what" question?

The "why" asks the question, why do I want to do this? Covey says that this question is the key to increasing your motivation. It helps us to walk through the fire and persevere. Here are several examples of "why" questions. "I'm exercising so that I can feel comfortable walking on the beach in my swimsuit." "I'm exercising so that my body image doesn't stop me from participating in certain activities." "I'm exercising so that I can feel a sense of accomplishment when my vision becomes a reality." What is *your* "why" question?

Finally, we get to the "how" question. This asks how I'm going to do it or what are that steps I'm going to take. You may answer this by saying, "I will start an exercise program that includes strength and cardiovascular training. Along with this I will change my nutritional patterns that may include cutting back on simple carbohydrates (or fats or calories), minimizing junk food and eating four to six small meals daily. Finally I will find someone who has accomplished goals similar to mine and ask this person for advice and encouragement." What is *your* "how" question?

Defining your goals in this way allows you to see that it's more than just saying, "What you want to do?" It's seeing a connection between why you want to do it and how you are going to do it and allowing this connection to begin motivating you to set the necessary goals.

> **What are your "what, why, and how" questions?**

Let's look at specific ideas you can use to make sure you accomplish your goals and eventually realize your vision.

1. Be sure to put your goal in writing

Putting your goal in writing helps you to clarify what you want to accomplish. When you write something on paper it makes you think about it more clearly. Once you've written it on paper be sure to put it in a spot where you will see it daily. If you remember back to Chapter 6, I suggested you do this as a reminder of your priorities. It works equally as well for goals. Don't forget it!

2. Each goal has to be specific

"I'm going to begin some aerobic activity." "I'm going to start eating better." "I will talk to someone about weight loss." These are not specific goals! You have to clearly define what it is you are going to do. Our example of losing 25 pounds for a vacation is a rather large goal and should be broken down incrementally, ultimately leading you toward weight loss.

> "**Important: Until you commit your goals to paper you have intentions that are seeds without soil.**"
> ~ **Anonymous**

I would set a series of small goals to create multiple success opportunities. Here are some examples.

- Exercise two times per week. That would include two strength training and two cardiovascular training segments. Later you can increase this.

- Increase your aerobic workout from 15 minutes to 20 minutes over a two-week period.

- Increase the weight you use on half of the strength training machines every third training session.

- Cut the amount of soda you drink from five cans per week to three cans.

Goals like this can be accomplished on a weekly basis. When you find yourself repeatedly accomplishing them you experience increased motivation because of your success. This initial motivation builds upon itself and grows, allowing you to achieve goal after goal, ultimately leading to accomplishment of your vision—in our example, the loss of 25 pounds.

3. Make the goals achievable

What you must never do is set unattainable goals. For instance, saying you are going to exercise six times per week for the next month when you haven't exercised six days in the last year is setting yourself up for failure. When you set up your goals, do so in a way that they require some effort, yet don't seem impossible. You don't want to be discouraged with failure after failure. By using the examples I previously mentioned you could expect reasonable success.

4. Set measurable goals

How do you know if you've accomplished a goal unless it's measurable? You can't! For example, if your goal is to look better in the mirror after the first month of exercise, you're setting an invitation for failure. How can you objectively measure this? Besides, what if you lose motivation before the first month is up? Then the goal can't be measured at all, even subjectively.

Let's look at the example goals I suggested in the section on "identifying specific goals." First, it's easy to measure whether or not you've exercised twice during the course of a week. All you have to do is mark off on a weekly calendar the days you exercised. Second, charting your progress in an exercise log makes it easy to see if you've increased your aerobic activity by five minutes in two weeks or to see if you've increased the weight you used on the strength training machines. Finally, keeping track of the number of cans of soda each week will tell you whether you were naughty or nice.

A measurable goal is going to give you proof of progress. This leads to greater motivation and greater motivation leads to success.

5. Put a time frame on your goal

In our example the time frame is to lose 25 pounds by the date of the vacation. You should even set time frames on each specific goal. The examples of specific goals I've been using have time frames attached to them. That is, increasing your aerobic activity by five minutes *in two weeks*, or adding weight to the strength training machines *every third session*. Also, you can say that for the first month of your exercise program you are going to exercise *two times per week*, then the second month you will increase to *three times per week* and so on.

Using time to help you achieve your goals can be very powerful. It serves as the stepping stone to the next level.

Take Action

It's easy to go through the work of creating your goals and preparing yourself to start something. However, it's another thing to get started. German poet and novelist Johann Wolfgang von Goethe once said, "Thinking is easy, acting is difficult, and to put one's thoughts into action is the most difficult thing in the world."

The greatest intent is useless unless you put it into action. Complacency will get you nowhere. A rocket requires 90% of its power at the initial thrust to get it moving into the air. The remaining 10% is all that's needed to keep it going. Take action today and start making progress toward achieving small goals that will ultimately lead to you realizing your vision.

> **"Thinking is easy, acting is difficult, and to put one's thoughts into action is the most difficult thing in the world."**
> ~ Goethe

Be Prepared for Change

There is no doubt some situation will arise that will throw a wrench in your plans. Suddenly, you get the flu and it sets you back two weeks in your exercise program. Or maybe your job requires you to travel and you can't find a decent place to work out. As a result, accomplishing two workouts a week becomes impossible. Or an old injury prevents you from progressing the way you had hoped.

Setbacks like these are very common. You can't let them halt your progress. Don't look at them as roadblocks, just detours. Based on the circumstances, you need to put together new goals that take into consideration the situation. If it's an injury that limits the amount of weight you can use on a particular strength-training machine, then find a different exercise that doesn't affect the injury. Maybe you can't find a good place to work out while on a business trip. Don't quit—do some crunches, push-ups, or rent an aerobic video.

Plan on things like this happening. Just don't give up. You're only a failure when you decide to quit.

Celebrate Your Success

The last thing to remember when setting your goals is to celebrate when you achieve them. I'm not just talking about the bigger goals, like losing 25 pounds for the vacation, but the smaller ones that are going to help get you there. You deserve it.

Take the time to spoil yourself. Buy yourself something. Get a massage. Do something that you wouldn't normally do. Rewarding yourself provides a little form of external motivation. Look forward to it and enjoy it.

Are You Following the Steps?

We've all set goals for one thing or another at some point in our lives. If I were to venture a guess, most people who set goals for exercise do not follow the steps I've just outlined. Statistics on exercise dropout rates prove my point.

If your barrier to exercise is a lack of motivation, take time to really think about why you are considering an exercise program. Create a vision. Make it real. You need to visualize yourself and how you will feel when it is accomplished. Then, start mapping out your goals that will serve as stepping-stones leading to your success with exercise.

Ninety-seven percent of people do not have a goals program simply because they do not know how to create one that works effectively. You are now one of the three percent who do. Take this knowledge and apply it to an exercise program.

As you start feeling the success associated with the achievement of each goal, you'll see your motivation will increase and you'll be on your way to making exercise a part of your life.

CHAPTER 8

Exercise Intimidates Me

What Causes Intimidation and How to Overcome It

"Anything I've ever done that ultimately was worthwhile initially scared me to death."
~ Betty Bender

This barrier to exercise is probably one of the most difficult to address. I say that because most of the issues surrounding intimidation are mental. Dealing with something you may have been feeling for months or even years can be very difficult, to say the least.

This is one of those unspoken barriers to exercise. It is not something that many people will openly admit. When I'm selling health club memberships to someone, they often use another excuse as to why they don't want to join rather than admitting they are too intimidated. To say you are intimidated to work out or join a health club can be embarrassing. It's saying that you are afraid. You are showing weakness. Nobody wants to admit that.

It seems society today tends to get hung up on a power trip. We want to be in control of our lives, not let someone control them. We want to have more money, more material things, a higher position in our company, and be the best at everything. People who are weak are looked down upon. So to admit that you feel intimidated to exercise out of fear, whether it is in a health club or at home, is something people tend to avoid.

As we talked about in Chapter 3, there are really only three places that you exercise—a health club, your home or outside.

Each of these places will bring with it a different intimidation factor, some more than others.

Intimidation tends to be a greater fear for those contemplating joining a health club. Therefore, most of what I say will be directed toward putting you at ease when it comes to exercising at a health club.

> **Intimidation tends to be a greater fear for those contemplating joining a health club.**

In addition, it's my opinion that a health club will, by far, give you the best environment to succeed with exercise. For those who are thinking of exercising at home, my advice will also be helpful; however, I don't see intimidation as an overriding barrier in that setting. The same is true for those who exercise outdoors.

In the previous chapter I discussed how important it is to have a vision and to use it as a weapon to achieve exercise success. When intimidation is a concern, having a vision can get you through. Remember that and dwell on these words by Charles Swindol, "With vision there is no room to be frightened. No reason for intimidation. It's time to march forward! Let's be confident and positive!" Let's march forward and overcome intimidation as a barrier to exercise.

Overcoming Intimidation

We will look into five variables that lead to feelings of intimidation when contemplating the start of an exercise program. As I mentioned earlier, these variables are heavily associated with a health club setting, but can also be relevant in other settings.

Age

Age can be a contributor to feelings of intimidation when it comes to physical activity. This can be a factor because you feel that you are unable to participate in an activity simply because you've hit a "magic number."

For example, say you're 55 years old and contemplating participation in a recreational sport. It could have been a sport you played when you were younger. However, when you look at others participating and see they are much younger, you say to yourself, "What was I thinking? I'm too old for this!" The result...no participation. I heard people make comments such as these even if they are fully capable of participating.

Another way age can be a factor is when you don't think you will fit in a particular setting because of your age. Many times this happens in conjunction with joining a health club. Health clubs get stereotyped as places where only young people exercise. Of course, this is a myth. Health clubs are for people of all ages. All you have to do is walk in one and find out. Now I will admit, there are specific times of the day when specific age groups have tendencies to work out. If age is an issue for you, visit the health club when people your age are working out.

Here are some statistics that the older readers may find comforting. According to a 2002 IHRSA/ASD Health Club Trend Report, 36% of the health club population consists of baby boomers (ages 35 to 54). This 36% represents approximately 12.9 million people, a 143% increase for this age group since 1987. Even more favorable for older adults is the increase of people over the age of 55 in health clubs across the country. In 2002, the 55 + age group accounted for 19% of the health club population. This represents a 42% increase in the last five years.

> **Fitness Fact**
>
> **Baby boomers represent 36% of the health club population.**

Get yourself going, jump on the bandwagon and follow the trend.

I think what it boils down to is how old you actually *feel*. I know people who are 60 years old and talk, act and function as though they are 80. Yet, you'll find people in their late 70s who are more vibrant and active than some in their 50s. Remember, age is just a number. You're only as old as you feel.

You can start an exercise program at any age. Just because you're 65 years old and never exercised a day in your life doesn't mean you can't start now. I have clients who didn't start any kind of weightlifting program until they were well in their 80s. Even at this age they made some fantastic progress. Now, there are some forms of exercise you may need to avoid for safety or medical reasons. You should consult with your physician before starting something new.

The truth is that you should never feel too old to start exercising. If you're looking for the fountain of youth, exercise is as close as it gets!

Fitness Level

There is no question that performing physical exercise can be difficult. To participate it takes energy, skill, physical ability and coordination. This scares the heck out of people. Many people feel they need to develop all this before they start an exercise program where other people are present.

So you're not in great shape, maybe you haven't exercised a day in your life. That's fine! You don't need to be in great shape to start an exercise program, just willing. Of the millions of people who exercise today, how many of them do you think started their exercise program in great shape? The answer is very few. Exercise was the tool that got them in great shape.

If your perceived fitness level is holding you back from exercise, here are some suggestions for you.

You will need to start slowly. Thinking you can't handle any type of exercise because you have a low fitness level is wrong. There are many activities that can help you increase your fitness level. Get out there and start walking or biking. Buy a treadmill. The key is to get started with something. You will never increase your level of fitness by sitting around thinking about it. Over the course of time you will be able to increase the difficulty of the activities you've chosen.

> "A year from now you may wish you had started today."
> ~ Karen Lamb

I would even suggest starting a light strength-training program right away. Believe me, you can do it. I have worked with many people who have never touched a weight machine in their lives get started and do just fine. In fact, many of them come back to me after only a few weeks and want to learn more. Don't make the assumption that something is too difficult unless you first give it a try.

What is important is that you begin slowly, and your fitness level will gradually improve through consistency and dedication. It won't be long and you will feel a wonderful increase in your stamina, strength, and self-esteem. At this point your level of fitness will no longer lead to feelings of intimidation.

Your Physique

This goes hand in hand with low fitness level. There is a good chance that if your fitness level isn't quite up to par then your physique probably doesn't look like a Greek statue. The way you view your body is one of the most common reasons for being intimidated. This is especially true when one is contemplating the start of an exercise program in the presence of others.

People who are overweight will often feel very apprehensive about getting started with exercise. Just because you are overweight does not mean you cannot begin to exercise. I've talked to people who actually think they need to get in shape or lose a few pounds before they join a health club. This type of thinking is absurd! Why do health clubs exist? They are there to get you started and help you in your quest to get in shape.

Don't think you need to have a great body to start exercise. A great physique is achieved only by taking the initiative to start an exercise program. You have to take the first step.

I have talked with enough people to know that it is hard to get over the feeling that others are looking at you. To be honest, people are more concerned with themselves than they are about looking at you. In fact, many people who you may think are looking at you were at some point in the same position you are. They are probably saying, "Good job, way to go for taking the first step."

Don't be concerned with what others are thinking. A majority of people aren't satisfied with their own body. What makes you think they are concerned with yours?

If your body still remains an issue, try exercising with a partner. Get a friend or family member to do it with you. When you exercise with a partner you get so caught up in conversation you won't even notice others around you.

For some, putting on a set of headphones and listening to their favorite music or book on tape helps them feel as ease.

Another popular trend today are "women-only" clubs. The reason these clubs were started was to eliminate the worry of being looked at by others, especially men. Women-only clubs cater to women who are overweight and feel too intimidated to join a regular health club. Could this be you?

If you are female and feel intimidated, women-only clubs can be a great way to get started. They provide a quick, full-body strength and cardiovascular workout in an exclusively female environment. However, I need to say something that may ruffle a few feathers, but many others and I feel is the truth. Women-only health clubs are a great way to get started, but after a while may become boring unless the club is set up like a regular health club. Here are my reasons for saying this.

Most women-only clubs are set up in a circuit style. That is, you go from machine to machine, with some very basic aerobic exercise mixed in, with each station being timed. The workout takes only a half hour and you are done. Sounds great, right? Well, almost.

The problem is that it doesn't take long for your body to adapt to this very simple stimulus, eventually leading to a decline in results. This decline is especially evident in long-term strength, endurance, and bone density improvements.

Cedric Bryant, vice president of educational services for the nonprofit American Council on Exercise, says, "The workout's benefits to an individual woman may begin to taper off with time. That's because the more fit a person is, the more vigorous and regular exercise they'll need to continue to see results. At some point they'll probably need to supplement it with other activities."

Bottom line, it may be a great way to start, but I would suggest moving on to something that will provide greater variety and an increasing level of difficulty.

Finally, if these options don't work for you, then at least get outside and find a quiet back road to use for walking or biking. Don't let your physique stop you from seeing what exercise can do in your life. After all, if you feel your body isn't what it should be, you owe it to yourself to get started.

Your Knowledge of Fitness

This is possibly the only legitimate reason to be intimidated by exercise. I can't even begin to count the number of magazines, books, self-proclaimed exercise gurus, and videos out there that are supposed to teach the proper ways to exercise. It can be very confusing! I can't believe the amount of fluff that is written today about exercise. It's seems like anybody can give themselves the title "fitness expert" and begin to disseminate information. Now don't get me wrong, there are many well-educated and knowledgeable people out there, but you need to be cautious.

Exercise is a science. In fact, my degree is in exercise science, so I can see how people get confused when trying to get started. This confusion leads to feelings of intimidation due to lack of knowledge. How many people will get involved with something they know nothing about? Not many! Nobody wants to look stupid!

> **Fitness Fact**
>
> **35% of people who hire a personal trainer do it for the motivation and education they receive.**
> **~ ACE poll**

If you feel lack of knowledge is the reason for your intimidation, don't give up. There are many reputable trainers that can help. I'm one of them! When you really need help building and properly executing an exercise program, my advice is to talk to a trainer one on one. They are more than willing to help you out. That's their job. They work with people like you all the time.

A recent poll conducted by the American Council on Exercise found that 35% of people who hire a personal trainer do so in order to get motivated and be educated on how to exercise properly. Take the time to find a trainer in your area.

If you are going to join a health club, many of them will provide you, free of charge, with a trainer who will show you the ropes and help you get started with a program that is based on your needs and goals. They are willing to answer all the questions you can throw at them. The beauty of a health club is that you have fitness professionals available at any time to help you.

If the health club setting isn't your thing, many personal trainers would be more than happy to go to your home and show you how to properly use the equipment you have available.

A trainer can help you with exercise regardless of where you choose to work out—at home, in a health club or anywhere. In a matter of several sessions, with a good trainer, you can figure on eliminating "lack of exercise knowledge" as a reason to be intimidated.

Socioeconomic status

Socioeconomic status isn't often an issue for people, but I wanted to comment on it because research shows this as an intimidation factor. I can't say that in my years of experience in this industry I've heard someone forgo exercise (in a health club) because they think it's a "status thing."

When I say "socioeconomic status," this is what I'm talking about. Some people will look at health or tennis clubs as places where only the wealthy or "the important people" choose to exercise. To some degree, a couple decades ago this may have been true, but not now. I see people from all walks of life join health clubs. It doesn't matter if you are the CEO of a Fortune 500 company or a bluecollar worker in a local factory; a health club is a welcoming place.

There is not a person on this planet that shouldn't be exercising. Whether you're rich or poor, the president of the United States or a hermit living in the mountains, you need to exercise. Socioeconomic status is not and should not be an issue.

So there you have them, the variables that contribute to intimidation and some ways to overcome them. Did one of them ring a bell? Maybe several struck a chord with you. I believe that most of your ability to overcome the obstacle of intimidation lies in your head. Psychologically, you need to get over the fear of intimidation.

It's Tough at First

Think back to the day when you took a new job or decided to take a night class at the local community college. I'll bet you felt a little uneasy or self-conscious, right? Maybe it had been years since you last opened a book that you actually had to study from. Then there is the thought of having to take tests again. This can be a scary time for you at first. However, it doesn't take long until you've developed some good study habits and realize that taking a test isn't that bad.

Joining a health club or starting an exercise program somewhere else is no different. At first you don't know anybody or are unsure of what to do, but within a short time you begin to feel more comfortable because you learn more each day and meet new people.

I once held a weight loss workshop for women only. At one of the sessions I asked, "What allowed you to get over the fear of exercising in a health club?" One of the women responded that she didn't worry what others were thinking and continued to be consistent with her exercise program. That meant day after day going into the gym and following her workout program. After a couple weeks she no longer had a fear of working out in the club when others were around. She soon made friends and realized that the people around her were all doing the same thing.

This is typical example and can work exactly the same way in your situation. Health clubs are not beauty pageants or places to go where you watch others. They are places where you can get professional help, use a variety of exercise equipment and have a great time socializing, all while getting in great shape.

What Are You Worth?

People who are intimidated by exercise, whether it's in a health club setting or anywhere, often are those who have low self-esteem. In many cases this comes from being overweight or in poor physical condition.

Nathaniel Brandon, a psychiatrist who studies self-esteem, says, "The nature of self-evaluation has a profound effect on a person's values, beliefs, thinking processes, feelings, needs, and goals." He goes on to say, "Self-esteem is the most significant key to a person's behavior."

Likewise, Brian Tracy, leading authority on personal and business success and bestselling author of 17 books, says, "Self-esteem precedes and predicts your performance in almost everything you do."

This concept can have a significant effect on whether or not you exercise. Many people who contemplate an exercise program face self-esteem issues. For some this becomes such a factor that it creates a barrier to exercise. Poet T.S. Eliot says, "Poor self-worth creates an invisible ceiling that can stop a person from attempting to rise above self-imposed limitations."

You cannot let your self-esteem stop you from starting an exercise program. Your thoughts control what you do, so if you constantly feed yourself with negative thinking about how you look, you will have real problems getting started.

> **"Poor self-worth creates an invisible ceiling that can stop a person from attempting to rise above self-imposed limitations."**
> ~ T. S. Eliot

In his best-selling book, *The Ultimate Weight Solution*, Dr. Phil McGraw (better known as Dr. Phil) talks about how many people will label themselves. He says, "Labels are self-descriptions in your internal dialogue that reflect certain conclusions you've reached about yourself."

The way you label yourself may come from past failures, the way people treated you, or cruel jokes that were aimed at you. When Dr. Phil writes about labeling he is referring to the labeling that goes on because of being overweight.

People in society who are overweight often get labeled. They hear things like: overweight people are lazy, have no willpower, and are unattractive. Is it right for people to do this? No, but it happens every day. And it will continue to happen.

Dr. Phil goes on to say, "Once you accept such a label as valid, you annihilate your self-confidence, your self-determination, and your longing for a healthier, more ideal weight."

You can't allow yourself to feel like this. It stifles any opportunity to get involved with exercise. So maybe you're overweight or out of shape. You'll always be like that unless you eliminate these feelings and get started. And that's just it, you have to start! The act of getting started will help replace these feelings with positive ones. The positive feelings come from the experiences you have with your own physical and mental changes and with the interaction of other people feeling the same thing.

It's amazing the number of people I speak with on a weekly basis who fear joining a health club for the reasons just cited. Their tone of voice, words, actions, and body gestures give it away. Whether you are working out in a health club or jogging down the street, you should be proud of what you are doing.

Rather than having feelings of intimidation and feeling like you're out of place, think of yourself as an inspiration to those who haven't taken the steps to start exercising. People who can't get themselves to exercise see you as an inspiration, someone to look up to. You may be the person who inspires them to begin an exercise program. Be proud of that. And for those people who are already participating in an exercise program, they look at you and think, "Welcome aboard! Good for you."

When you are finally able to conquer intimidation as a barrier to exercise you will wonder why it was an issue to begin with. You'll begin to see how exercise will improve your life physically, mentally, and emotionally.

The newfound self-confidence that comes from greater self-esteem will equip you to handle the stress and daily challenges you face and become a stronger, more successful person.

The small step you take to overcome this barrier to exercise will have a lasting impact on your life. You will become a better, more positive person who can change other people's lives as well. You owe it to yourself to feel this way. Something as simple as exercise can be the catalyst to making this a reality.

CHAPTER 9

I Find Exercise Boring

Inspiring Ways to Make Exercise Enjoyable for You

"A pessimist sees the difficulty in every opportunity; an optimist sees the opportunity in every difficulty."
~ Winston Churchill

If you've read this far, you already realize that variety is a great antidote to boredom. For some specific suggestions, I took the liberty to interview a number of members at my health club. I chose members who have demonstrated consistency with working out over the years. These are people that have made exercise a part of their lives. When choosing whom to interview I selected people of different ages, fitness goals, and physical conditions.

The first question I asked was whether or not they found exercise to be enjoyable. I also wanted to find out why they chose to exercise. I feel that knowing why you are doing something goes a long way toward determining whether you will be consistent as well as successful.

There is power in the testimonials you are going to read because they came from real people who are in the same boat as you. This is not theoretical information derived from a textbook on how to make exercise enjoyable. These people offer insight on how they make exercise enjoyable enough to incorporate into their lifestyle.

Testimonial #1

Name: Jean
Age: 45
Occupation: Mother of 3
Years of Exercise: 2

"When I decided to start an exercise program, I did it because I wanted to lose some weight and get my body in shape so I could feel good about myself. I'm one of those people that actually find exercise enjoyable. With it comes a sense of accomplishment; it fuels my desire to stay in shape. I have a personal trainer that works with me several days a week and keeps it interesting. Some days I'll walk on the treadmill, lift weights, ride a bike or work on my flexibility. It's always different. I can honestly say that I enjoy exercise."

> **"It's enjoyable for me because of the variety of exercises I have to choose from."**
> **~ Jean**

Testimonial #2

Name: Dave
Age: 39
Occupation: Realtor
Years of Exercise: 10

"I am a 39-year-old father of three very active kids ages 2, 4, and 8. I want to be able to keep up with my kids when they are in high school and not be a dad that just sits around. In addition, exercise makes me feel more alert and allows me to be successful in my career. When working out I usually do some type of aerobic activity like the treadmill or elliptical trainer. Between these machines I'll spend an hour, four or five days a week. I would have to say that having TVs to watch while on the machines really makes it easy to

> **"I would have to say having TVs to watch while on the machines really makes it easy to work out for this length of time."**
> **~ Dave**

work out for this length of time. Since I got going on this routine it hasn't been a problem keeping up with it on a daily basis. I look forward to it."

Testimonial #3

Name: Phil
Age: 54
Occupation: Licensed Practical Nurse
Years of Exercise: 7

"Is exercise enjoyable or boring? I would have to say both. At times I feel it gets a little stale. During these times I continue to do it because I know it's good for me. Heck, we don't eat peas because we like them; we eat them because they are good for us! My workouts consist mainly of lifting weights and playing ice hockey in the winter with the kids I coach. Exercise, for me, is an opportunity to get away from things. I also see it as a way to keep in shape, so as I get older, I can continue to play golf, volleyball, and waterski. Most of the time I do find exercise enjoyable; however, there are weeks when I get bored with it. During these times I think of all the reasons I'm doing it and it keeps me going."

> **"Exercise, for me, is an opportunity to get away from things."**
> **~Phil**

Testimonial #4

Name: Curt
Age: 41
Occupation: Welder
Years of Exercise: 12

"For the most part I would have to say that I find exercise to be enjoyable. There are, however, times when I get bored with it. I overcome that boredom by the very fact that I've developed a sense of

> **"I overcome that boredom by the very fact that I've developed a sense of routine from it in my life."**
> **~Curt**

routine from it in my life. This routine drives me through those days when I don't feel like working out. I mainly get involved with lifting weights. Through this I find a sense of relief from all the stress I undergo. In addition, I find exercise to be enjoyable because I *can* exercise. The rush that comes along with exercise and the ability to do it keeps me going back for more."

Testimonial #5

Name: Jill
Age: 44
Occupation: Bank Teller
Years of Exercise: 2

"I have to say it took me a little while before I actually enjoyed exercise. What really makes it fun for me is the socializing that comes along with it. I have a friend who exercises with me most of the time. We chitchat while walking on the treadmill or using the elliptical trainer. Time passes quickly. I started exercising because I had a number of health issues that required me to take a lot of medications. I didn't like it and wanted a change! I am happy to say that after nine months I am off all medications. There are times when I find it difficult to get to the gym and exercise. Sometimes I don't feel like getting up in the morning or it's too cold outside and don't feel like getting in my car to drive to the gym. In times like this I'm thankful I have somebody to exercise with like my trainer or my friend. When I know they are at the gym waiting for me, I don't want to let them down."

> **"What really makes it fun for me is the socializing that comes along with it."**
> ~Jill

Testimonial #6

Name: Elaine
Age: 65
Occupation: Recently retired nurse
Years of Exercise: 3

"I started exercising because I wanted to get rid of all my aches and pains. I first tried exercising at home, but that didn't work.

So I thought I would try the local health club. After three years of consistent exercise I can truly say that I enjoy it. I enjoy the fact that I am now feeling better and have no more backaches or stiffness. It's

> "Believe it or not, the fact that I am paying a monthly membership fee keeps me exercising."
> ~Elaine

great! What makes exercise enjoyable for me is the variety of exercises to choose from and having a professional trainer help me whenever I get confused. Believe it or not, the fact that I am paying a monthly membership fee keeps me exercising as well. After all, I don't want to waste my money. Lastly, I enjoy the male and female atmosphere the health club has to offer. It makes things more enjoyable."

I really enjoyed talking with these people about what exercise meant to them. We all can learn from what they had to say. To see each person's perspective on exercise was very encouraging.

During the interview process I didn't find one person who said exercise was boring and a waste of time. Now I'm sure there are people out there that are bored to death with exercise. You may be one of them! Over the years I've been in contact with people like this. However, one common denominator among those who find exercise enjoyable is years of experience with exercise. It's enjoyable to them because they know what works and what doesn't and they've experienced the improved quality of life it brings.

Exercise With Value

When you read through the testimonials earlier in the chapter you'll see there is some commonality among each of them. It's not so much the fact that they like the physical act of exercise, rather the value it brings to their lives. It was the value they saw in exercise that allowed them to overcome the boredom. They've been able to experience the joy that exercise brings, not only in their lives, but also the lives of those around them. In addition, these people didn't look only at the immediate appeal exercise brings, such as weight loss, self-confidence, or better muscle tone; but how it will effect their longevity, that is their ability to keep up as they get older. This is especially true if they have young kids. Keeping up with them as they get older is important and perceived as valuable. For some, exercise is important because they see it as a means to continue enjoying the same recreational activities later in life that they enjoy now.

When I asked, "Do you enjoy exercise?" and most of them answered "yes," it wasn't for the sheer love of sweat and hard work, but the value they new it would bring. Dr. Martin Luther King once said, "The quality, not the longevity, of one's life is what is important." You need to look

> **You need to look beyond the short-term discomfort and see the lasting joy exercise can bring to your life.**

beyond the short-term discomfort and see the lasting joy and quality it can bring to your life. The people I interviewed see that value.

For the remainder of this chapter, I would like to help you find a way to enjoy exercise immediately, so that you can stick with it and become one who finds exercise truly enjoyable long-term as well.

We will look at some ways to figure out what type of exercise you enjoy, how to make traditional exercise more interesting and how you can turn your normal day-to-day activities into meaningful exercise.

Using Exercise History to Make It Work

You may think the idea of perceived value is great for some people, but it doesn't work for you. That's okay. If this is the case we need to look at another way to overcome exercise boredom.

Think back to a time when you participated in a physical activity that you enjoyed. Surely, you can think of something at some point in your life you liked. It may have been a recreational activity such as volleyball, basketball, or softball. Maybe while in high school or college you were active in a sport that you really enjoyed. How about a time when you got together with a friend or group of friends and went walking, biking, or cross-country skiing on a regular basis? Take some time to think back and figure out what type of physical activity you enjoyed in the past.

Now let's look at some questions and solutions for bringing back this type of exercise into your life.

1.   What activity was it that you enjoyed?

2.   What did you like most about it?

3.   Who were the people that made it enjoyable?

4.   Where were you most likely to participate in this activity?

5.   Why did you like it?

My hope is that some of these questions jogged your memory, no pun intended! Now I'm sure some of the things that made this activity enjoyable are impossible to relive; however, by bringing back some of the elements you can get started again.

For example, maybe you frequently participated in local marathons or short races at a younger age. You remember most of your training for the race was done after work and just before supper. It made you feel good, like your day was complete. In addition, a friend would often join you for a workout, making it a pleasant experience.

At this point you may be saying there is no way I am going to train like I did for the marathon or other race, let alone run one. I'm not saying that you need to run a marathon again. My point is that you should look for the elements that made it enjoyable. Think back a little. You had a regular workout time that made you feel good. If this time will again work in your life, then go for it. Also, part of the reason you liked the workout was because a friend joined you. Get together with that same friend. If you've lost touch with that person, then ask a new friend to come along.

The point I am making is that you need to find out why you liked and regularly participated in exercise before, and bring those elements into your life now. Hey, it worked then, why not now?

If you can't remember any type of exercise you enjoyed, then take a look at the next section and see if any of these ideas will work.

Is This Really Exercise?

Before we get too involved with this section, I want to briefly reiterate what makes up a complete exercise program. Exercise should consist of three parts: cardiovascular (aerobic) exercise, strength training and flexibility, as mentioned in Chapter 3.

It is very important to include all three of these components in your routine. Many people associate exercise with only cardiovascular activity such as walking, jogging, biking or aerobic tapes. This form of exercise is not complete without the other components.

Now, for those of you who absolutely object to the thought of a regular exercise program, this is for you. Below you will find some ways to make your everyday activities into meaningful exercise. I don't recommend this as your only exercise because nothing can replace a complete exercise program, but this will help you become more active.

> ## Truth vs. Myth
>
> **Myth: A physically demanding job can take the place of exercise.**
>
> **Truth: True exercise includes cardiovascular, strength and flexibility training.**

1. Enjoy more time with your children

Kids are some of the most active creatures on the planet! My three-year-old keeps me going from the minute I get home from work until bedtime. He is a bundle of energy.

For those of you who have young kids, you know what I'm talking about. Kids and physical activity are synonymous. Get out there and play catch or tag, go biking, take hikes through the woods or splash around in the water with them. The things you can do are endless. If you are at a loss for things to do, just ask your kids. They will find something to do.

Even if your kids are older and past the "playing" stage, get together with them and go for a walk or bike ride. Maybe you can participate in a recreational sport together or a hobby that requires physical activity. Not only are you more active, but you're also spending some great quality time with those who mean the most in your life.

2. Get active at work

The first thing you can do is park a little further away from your office. Heck, you can do this even when shopping. Don't always look for the closest parking spot. A fringe benefit to this is that you don't have to look hard for a spot or worry about the driver of the car next to you denting your car.

Also, take the stairs rather than an elevator. Stair climbing is an excellent form of exercise. Taking stairs throughout the course of the day equals extra calories expended. According to healthstatus.com, in the minute it may take you to stand in the elevator you can burn up to eight times more calories walking up the stairs.

Occasionally, when you aren't in a hurry, rather than calling

> **Get some exercise at work by turning a small meeting into "walking and talking.**

someone in your office building on the phone to ask a question, go to their office and ask them person-ally. Not only does this provide an opportunity to exercise, but a chance to visit. If this is inconven-ient, simply standing while you're on the phone will burn more calories than sitting.

How about turning a small meeting into an exercise session by "walking and talking?" This probably won't work with large groups; however, when only a few of you have things to discuss it may be a perfect opportunity to move around. Studies show improved brain functioning when you are physically active. Walking and talking may stir up your creativity!

3. Find a hobby that keeps you active

The list of hobbies can be endless when you think about it. You can go hiking, canoeing, rock climbing, gardening, water-skiing, cross-country skiing, birdwatching, rollerblading, golfing, play tennis or badminton, hunting, and on and on. If you are wondering how many calories various activities expend, go to www.healthstatus.com or www.diabetes.about.com. These websites have a large variety of activities to choose from.

Getting involved in a hobby where you can be outdoors with friends or family can be very rewarding. You may even forget that you are exercising.

4. Combine fitness with your family chores

> ### Fitness Fact
> ___
> **Even gardening can burn up to 323 calories per hour!**

I know doing chores is not an activity most people enjoy. Furthermore, having to do these things cuts down on your available time to exercise. However, they need to get done. How about making some of these chores into exercise?

You can rake leaves instead of using the lawnmower to pick them up. Lois Sheldahl, director of the cardiopulmonary rehabilitation unit at the Veterans' Affairs Medical Center in Milwaukee, looked at the amount of energy it takes to perform various household tasks. She found that raking could burn up to 5.75 calories per minute. That's almost 200 calories in just over 30 minutes of raking!

Landscaping can be very physical if you have to haul dirt, sand and rocks to different areas of your yard.

If you own a fireplace you need to have wood for burning. Instead of buying it, find a place where you can cut it down yourself. Or, have the person who delivers it throw it into a big pile, so you will have to stack it.

> ### F.Y.I.
> ___
> **Mowing lawn with a push mower can burn up to eight calories a minute.**

For many people, cutting the lawn is a weekly chore. Instead of using your riding lawnmower (men, I know this will be hard), use a push mower. It can be fantastic exercise, especially if you have a big yard.

Some of you are probably thinking I'm crazy to suggest these things. Why make the chores harder than they already are? Remember, you don't have to do this if you get involved in a regular exercise program. Ask yourself, what is the lesser of two evils? The whole idea is to get more active and this is one way to do it.

Put Some Spark in Traditional Exercise

Does your current workout go something like this? You drag yourself to the gym, waste some time getting into your workout clothes in order to prolong the monotonous task of walking on the treadmill. Finally you're dressed and you manage to make it to the treadmill section. You get on and reluctantly set the timer for 30 minutes. Five minutes hasn't even gone by and you're already bored out of your mind. You think to yourself, "I've only been doing this for a couple weeks and I'm already sick of it, how can I make it a lifestyle?"

Can you relate to this scenario? We are creatures of habit. Whether we start the day by reading the morning newspaper or watching a particular television program each week, we tend to form patterns that are hard to break. When it comes to exercise, patterns may be counterproductive as boredom sets in. Many people can get stuck in this rut if they don't know how to make traditional exercise more interesting.

When you are thinking of beginning a more traditional style exercise program, you need to ask yourself a few questions. These questions will help you to make the activity more enjoyable and rewarding.

Do you want to be social or would you rather exercise by yourself?

If you want to be social, then join a health club! There is no better place to meet and talk with people with similar interests than a health club. At a club you can attend an aerobic or other type of group training class. Don't be afraid if you've never tried one before; many clubs will have introductory classes to help you get started. The atmosphere in a group class is exciting, exhilarating and filled with variety. In addition, people who get involved with group exercise tend to have a stronger commitment to exercise than when exercising individually.

If a group class is not what you are interested in, then take advantage of the other equipment a club has to offer. The variety of the equipment alone is worth the membership dues. I highly recommend mixing up your workout with various machines and equipment on a regular basis. One of the people I interviewed for a testimonial at the beginning of this chapter stated that it is the variety of equipment she uses that makes exercise fun. I truly believe this is the key to making exercise work for you. It works in two ways. First, you will find exercise more enjoyable because of the variety of equipment. Second, the variety will also help you see faster and more long-lasting results.

> ## Fitness Fact
>
> ---
>
> **People who get involved with group exercise tend to have a stronger commitment to exercise than when exercising individually.**

If the social atmosphere is the last thing you want and would like to exercise by yourself, then I would suggest a home gym or exercising outdoors.

A home gym can offer a fair amount of variety. This, however, comes with a higher up-front price tag. The more variety you want, the more you have to spend. Refer to Chapter 10 for details on costs and options. If you don't like to be around other people when you exercise, this is the way to go. You need to ask yourself, "How much is my health worth?"

Another option for exercising by yourself is to go outside for a walk, a bike ride or a swim. As mentioned earlier, there are many outdoor recreational activities to choose from. To some degree it depends on where you live in the country. You can participate in most outdoor activities by yourself. They are called silent sports.

Now, as I mentioned previously, outdoor activities only encompass one or two components of exercise, those components being cardiovascular and flexibility training. When exercising exclusively outdoors you are missing the strength-training component.

While many people prefer exercising on their own, consider this point. Studies have shown that long-term adherence to exercise diminishes when you exercise by yourself. This doesn't mean that it won't work if you choose to exercise alone. However, the odds are against you. That choice is up to you. You need to consider the good and bad of each and determine what will help you be most successful with exercise.

Do you want to get energized with your workout or wind down?

For some people a good workout can energize them, while others get tired and are ready for a nap. Everybody is different. The point of this question isn't what you feel like after the workout, but how you want to feel during the workout.

For those of you who are looking to get energized, pumped up and excited while exercising, you need to do some type of aerobic class or lift weights. As I mentioned in the last section, an aerobic class or any other cardiovascular activity will get your heart pumping and that is what you want to do—get your heart pumping! Too many people hop on a treadmill and walk at a pace that hardly stimulates the heart. Get moving!

> **When it comes to aerobic activity—get your heart pumping!**

There are even aerobic classes that combine aerobic activity with a strength segment. Wow, the best of both worlds!

Strength training with free weights can be an awesome experience. Feeling the pump in the muscles, seeing your strength increase and knowing that with each workout you are going to look better leads to an energizing experience. All you ladies out there need to realize that strength training isn't just for men. More and more women are getting involved and realizing that exercise is more than just participating in aerobic activity.

Now we come to the second half of the question: do you want to exercise to help wind down? For some the thought of going through an aerobics class and jumping around is not what they're looking for after a long day at work. Or, maybe you have a physical job and can't bear the thought of lifting weights when the day is done. For many people these are legitimate concerns. So you're probably thinking, "Oh good, I've got an excuse not to exercise." Wrong!

Right now there are classes becoming very popular across the country that may be just right for you. I'm talking about yoga, Pilates or tai chi. What a great way to wind down your day and get a good dose of exercise in the process.

Yoga is more popular today than ever before. There are various styles of yoga ranging from powerful and intense to soothing and relaxing. The benefits include increased muscular endurance, balance and flexibility to skeletal alignment, rehabilitation and stress relief depending on the style of yoga you choose.

> **Fitness Fact**
> _____
>
> **The fastest growing exercise forms tend to be workouts that are less taxing...the top growth activity was Pilates.**

Pilates emphasizes the uniform development of all muscle groups while in the process promoting flexibility, circulation and skeletal alignment. The abdominal region is the main focus along with emphasis on the back and upper leg musculature. According to the 2002 Superstudy of Sports Participation conducted by American Sports Data, Inc., Pilates was the top growth activity in the fitness industry in 2001.

Tai chi is considered a moving form of yoga and meditation combined. It can enhance balance, flexibility, gait, posture, digestion, concentration, memory and overall physical and mental well-being.

Are you a goal-oriented person or do you want to be flexible?

When you ask yourself this question, I hope you say that you are more goal-oriented. I truly believe that a goal-orientated person will be more successful with exercise. It's really tough to stay with exercise if you are doing a little of this and a little of that with no real goal or reason in mind.

It's likely that the first couple months of exercise will yield good results. If you're still with it at this time, further results become difficult. This is true because the body adapts and does-n't need to change.

"The human body is very good at adapting to the stresses it experiences," says Lisa Packheiser, a certified athletic trainer. "Performing the same activity repeatedly at the same level makes the body more efficient, which eventually results in lower caloric expenditure from the activity. In fact, research shows that by sticking to just one activity, the number of calories burned by exercisers may decrease by as much as 25%." Having various goals helps you to focus and make the necessary changes.

I do, however, believe that being flexible can make it easier to exercise because you are not tied down to a mundane routine. You should note that being goal-oriented doesn't necessarily mean you can't be flexible.

If you are a goal-oriented person, any type of exercise will work for you. The key is to make sure you know what your goals are. We discussed this in Chapter 7. Create a vision and from this vision you can establish goals that will be used to monitor progress toward seeing the vision become a reality.

You need to chart and monitor your progress. Do this by having a workout log. It can be used for charting your aerobic activity, weight training, outdoor

> ## Training Tip
>
> ---
>
> **Charting will allow you to see improvement on a weekly basis. Seeing this improvement on paper will create excitement. This excitement leads to enjoyment.**

activities, or group classes like yoga and Pilates. Charting will allow you to see improvement on a weekly basis. Seeing this improvement on paper will create excitement. This excitement leads to enjoyment.

On the other hand, if you are not goal-oriented and want to be flexible with your exercise, you can still see results. The results you see may be more sporadic and less noticeable without goals to mark your progress. That's okay. You are what you are and if you want to be flexible then so be it.

I would recommend that regardless of what exercises you choose, write them down. Use this information the next time you exercise to take it one step further. For example, if one day you decide to strength train the chest and arms (also known as the beach workout), make sure you write down how much weight you lifted along with the number of sets and repetitions you did so that the next time you work out you can increase the effort. Increase effort by adding weight, sets or changing the reps.

If you choose to be flexible from week to week and do not have any real goals or scheduled exercises in your routine, that is fine providing it works for you. It can work to your benefit because you are doing what you want to do whenever you want to do it. This can make it interesting. Just beware that you should incorporate each component (i.e., cardiovascular, strength and flexibility training) each week. It is also important that as you spontaneously choose what you want to do, be sure to work each muscle group regularly and chart the progress you make.

Master the Art of Distraction

If you find exercise boring, regardless of what type you do or where you choose to do it, then you need to distract yourself. There are several ways you can do this.

If you spend a lot of time walking on a treadmill, riding a bike or using an elliptical trainer, I would suggest you utilize some form of entertainment while sweating away the calories. You can do this by purchasing a portable CD or cassette player and listen to your favorite music. You can even listen to books on tape. For those of you who are "techies," you probably have an mp3 player that can hold hundreds of songs or books in one small unit. Just download the material from your computer to the mp3 player and you have an instant distraction. I know many people in my health club who do this. If this is too technical for you then go the old-fashioned route. Bring in a book or magazine to read while exercising. People do it all the time. Most exercise equipment will have a holder for your book so it is convenient to read.

Training Tip

Distract yourself by listening to music or books on tape, watch TV, surf the Web, or find a friend to exercise with.

Whether you are at home or in a health club you can exercise while watching television. Most clubs have entertainment centers where you can listen to the sound on the television through your own set of headphones. Why not watch your favorite program while walking on the treadmill instead of sitting in the recliner eating popcorn.

More and more health clubs are attaching small computer screens with Internet access to their cardiovascular equipment. Just think, you can surf the Web and e-mail your friends while walking on a treadmill. Heck, you can even shop for gifts while exercising by going to a website and having your purchases shipped directly to your home. Only in the 21st century!

Finally, find a friend to exercise with. Study after study has shown that exercise is more enjoyable and rewarding when you have a friend to do it with. It makes the time go more quickly and you can help each other if any exercise-related questions arise.

Realize the Rewards

You would think the simple fact of knowing exercise helps prevent heart disease, some forms of cancer, diabetes, obesity and other health-related problems would be enough for someone to exercise regularly. Unfortunately this knowledge alone doesn't do it.

People who successfully incorporate exercise into their lifestyle have done so by following the examples outlined in this chapter. But even more than practicing what I've discussed, people who exercise regularly do it because they see

"I asked for all things, that I might enjoy life. God gave life, that I might enjoy all things."
~Unknown author

the rewards it brings. Some of these rewards are immediate and some are yet to be realized.

Take time to read over the testimonials at the beginning of this chapter again. They are people just like you who have made exercise a lifestyle, not necessarily because they love to do it, but because of what it does for them. You can't put a price tag on your health and the ability to play with your children or participate in your favorite hobby or activity. Dwell on this fact and apply the knowledge you've learned in this chapter to help you overcome exercise boredom.

CHAPTER 10

I Can't Afford to Exercise

How Much it Really Costs and Ways to Make It Work for You

"Lack of money is no obstacle. Lack of an idea is an obstacle."

~Ken Hakuta

Money! Now that is a touchy subject, especially during times of economic distress. With 80% of the nation's wealth controlled by only 20% of the population, I'm going to guess you probably don't have an overabundance of money.

Paying bills each month can be a dreadful activity. For some even the ring of the telephone can cause a heartbeat to skip out of fear it is a creditor asking for their money. Then there are the times when your car breaks down or the furnace goes out in your house. "Where am I going to get the money to pay for that?" you cry. A large number of people in this country live paycheck to paycheck. Then there is that evil piece of plastic called a credit card. Sixty percent of Americans do not pay off their credit cards each month. This has resulted in $660 billion in credit card debt.

For many people this is reality. There just doesn't seem to be enough money each month to pay the bills. If you're in this situation, then I'm sure you

> ### Frightening Fact
>
> **Sixty percent of Americans do not pay off their credit cards each month, resulting in $660 billion in credit card debt.**

think spending money on starting an exercise program is the last thing you need. Right? Wrong!

I'm not a financial expert nor do I aspire to be one. There are many great financial counselors available and books on the market for you to choose from. In fact, a book that I found very helpful is the *Total Money Makeover: A Proven Plan to Financial Fitness*, by Dave Ramsey. It's a life-changing book that has some wonderful techniques you can begin immediately.

Since I'm not a financial guru, what I intend to do in this chapter is explain to you the costs involved with starting an exercise program, how easy it is to waste money on things that can be budgeted toward exercise, and finally, some inexpensive ways to get started.

Now, if you are fortunate to have money that can be put toward starting an exercise program, good for you. You earned it. I would suggest you skip to the final chapter.

For those of you who are struggling, read on.

How Much Does It Really Cost?

As I've mentioned earlier in the book, there are several ways you can start an exercise program. You can exercise outside, buy equipment for your home, or join a health club. Let's take a look at some price breakdowns for each.

Enjoying the great outdoors

By now you've realized the most inexpensive route is to start a program that involves outdoor activity such as walking, jogging or swimming. If you already own a bike, which most people do, you can start biking on a regular basis. There are other outdoor activities to choose from if you have the equipment, including cross-country skiing, snowshoeing, canoeing or rollerblading. You can join a basketball, volleyball, or soccer team that plays indoors or outdoors for year-round exercise. Many people already own the equipment—it just needs to be used.

Start small at home

The next most inexpensive way to start exercising is to buy some aerobic tapes, small dumbbells, and exercise tubing or fitness balls for your home. These items are fairly inexpensive, ranging in price from $4 for exercise tubing to $15 to $25 for an aerobic tape. You can even buy videos showing you how to use the exercise tubing and fitness balls. For around $50 you can get a fitness ball, exercise tubing and a video showing you how to use them. If you really want to get started on a low budget, this is the way to go. However, I need to warn you that after several months you will need a change in order to continue seeing results. By this time you will probably have seen the positive impact exercise has made in your life and will be ready to go to the next level.

F.Y.I.
_____

For around $50 you can get a fitness ball, exercise tubing and a video showing you how to use them.

Progress to a health club

Where you live will determine the cost of joining a health club. According to the International Health, Racquet and Sportsclub Association, the median cost to join a health club in 2002 was $55 per month. This takes into account the very high-priced clubs and the lowest priced clubs. I've seen clubs range in price from $19 a month to $100-plus a month. There really is quite a range.

F.Y.I.
_____

The median cost to join a health club is about $55 per month. However, this can vary greatly.

If you live in smalltown America then you are probably looking at paying somewhere in the upper $30s to low $40s per month. For example, I live in a town of approximately six thousand people and as of 2004 our monthly rate for a regular membership is $39, with limited memberships starting at $29.99 per month. Some of the big-name clubs will run promotions where you can get in for only $19 a month.

Now, you must also know that you will probably have to pay an initiation or enrollment fee at most clubs. These are one-time fees paid upon joining. They can range from no fee at all to $200.

Think about it, for as little as $19 per month you get a huge variety including both strength and cardiovascular training equipment. On top of that you get a professional trainer to design and guide you through a program made just for you. If you ask me, that's a steal.

Going bigger at home

When you think about buying home gym equipment on a larger scale you are probably looking at a higher up-front cost. What I'm saying is that most of the time you will purchase a piece of equipment and pay for it in full. Although in this day and age of credit, many companies will finance the equipment for you so you can make monthly payments. If you go this route watch out for the interest rate.

Exercise equipment for your home can have a wide price range depending on what you want. Below I've listed some of the price ranges for cardiovascular equipment.

Stationary bikes—$ 200–$500
Treadmills—$200–$8,000
Rowing machines—$200–$3,500
Cross-country ski machines—$300–$750
Stair steppers—$50–$3,000
Elliptical trainers—$300–$3,800

As you can see there is a wide range in the pricing. For the most part, the upper end of pricing is more representative of commercial quality equipment. If you and your family will be the only ones using the equipment, then a commercial unit would be overkill.

Strength training equipment can also have a wide price range depending on what you get. You can go as simple as some dumbbells for $4 a pair, as I mentioned earlier, or you can buy a multi-station strength training machine ranging in price from

$250 to $5,500. Generally speaking, the higher the price the more exercise options you get on the machine.

If you don't want to buy something brand new then you can consider a pre-owned piece of equipment. Check your local newspaper or stores that sell used equipment. However, make sure you see the equipment before agreeing to buy it. Safety should be your number one concern.

Finding Money for Exercise?

Now that you are up-to-date on the costs involved with starting an exercise program, let's look at how Americans spend money. I want you to see how much money you can save and put toward exercise by just making some minor adjustments in your spending habits. Some of this may come as a surprise to you.

Cigarette smoking is the number one preventable cause of death in the United States today. Close to one million people lose their lives each year due to cigarette smoking. Wow! If this isn't bad enough, look at how much money is spent on cigarettes. Let's say you smoke one pack of cigarettes a day at a cost of roughly $5 a pack. When you do the math that equals $150 per month or $1,800 per year spent on smoking. I'm not going to give you a lecture on why you should

> ### Frightening Fact
> ─────────────
> **Smoking just one pack of cigarettes a day can cost you nearly $1,800 a year!**

quit smoking; however, if you are a smoker you need to wake up and smell the coffee! This is money that can be spent towards exercise or something else of value. Even if you cut your smoking habit by 25% you can afford a health club membership or some home gym equipment.

Another way to save money to put towards exercise is to go out to eat less frequently. Whether it is fast food for lunch or going out for supper, it adds up. Your average fast food meal will cost you from $4 to $5. If you go out just two times a week it will cost you almost $40 a month. I know people who eat at a fast food restaurant four times a week. What would it take for you to pack a lunch a couple days a week and save the money? It would certainly be more nutritious.

If you frequently go out for supper it will cost you even more. The average bill for a dinner at a mid-priced restaurant can range from $9 to $15 plus drinks. If you only go out once a week for supper with a spouse or significant other you can expect to spend up to $35. Depending on where you live in the country, going out for a nice dinner can cost a whole lot more.

Again, I'm not saying that you shouldn't go out to eat, just cut back a little. Even cutting back just once a week will save you enough money to join most health clubs.

You would be surprised at how the little things can add up. Drinking one cup of gourmet coffee a day from your favorite coffee house costs you $450 or more a year. Those of you who love to drink soda spend $275 a year if you only drink one per day. One per day, that's nothing. I know people who drink a six-pack daily! If you like to buy magazines off the rack to the tune of one per week, expect to part with $150 each year.

F.Y.I.

Cut back your spending by just $10 a week and you can join many health clubs or buy equipment for your home.

The list of small items goes on and on. Things like lottery tickets, video rentals, books, newspapers, or treats for the kids all add up. How about when you are in the convenience store to pay for gas and you pick up a few extra (higher priced) items like candy, milk, pizza or pastries?

If you take time to stop and think about the money you spend on a regular basis for the small items I've just mentioned, you see that there is a lot of opportunity to save. The beauty is that it doesn't take much. A little here and a little there will go a long way. Cutting back by just $10 a week can buy you a health club membership or some simple exercise equipment for your home. What is $10 a week? Two packs of cigarettes, a couple fast food meals or a few bottles of soda? Not much! I challenge you to take a look at your spending habits and see how easy it can be to afford something that is good for you...like exercise.

How Important Is
Your Health to You?

I want to close this chapter with a story about a client I once had who found a way to make exercise work.

For the sake of anonymity we will call her Jane. Jane was a massage therapist who didn't make a whole lot of money. In addition to her massage therapy she spent time as a waitress in the evening and on weekends to help make ends meet. She was not married, so didn't have a second income in the household.

She was approaching her 50th birthday and had been active in the past but couldn't be consistent with it. Knowing that she wasn't getting any younger she wanted to stay active with some consistency. But to do it on her own was too difficult.

Since she was a massage therapist at a local health club she was fortunate to receive free membership at the club. Certainly this was a great fringe benefit. With this benefit, cost was not an issue; however, getting motivated to exercise was. She thought about hiring a personal trainer but knew it would cost her over $20 a session. But, if she wanted to be consistent she knew she would have to work out with a trainer at least two times per week. This would cost her over $160 a month. In her mind she thought that would be too difficult to handle.

After a lot of thought and prioritizing she agreed to hire a personal trainer. She worked out twice a week every week for nearly three years. She made some fantastic improvements in her strength, stamina, body composition and overall health. In fact, she had her bone density measured and it was 110% of the norm for a woman her age! It changed her life.

The point I want to make with this story is that she found a way to pay for the services of a personal trainer. Instead of spending all her tip money from massage therapy and the restaurant, she put it in a jar to save for her training sessions. She paid each week with cash. I'm sure it took Jane some discipline to save the money; however, it was well worth it.

You can't put a price tag on your health. Most people don't realize how valuable it is until it's gone. The thought of making a few adjustments in your spending habits seems trivial compared to difficulties faced when your health is falling apart due to neglect.

Henry Ford said, "The highest use of capital is not to make more money, but to make money do more for the betterment of life." Most likely Ford was talking about the money used to build cars that would ultimately improve the quality of life. Which it did! However, you can take this quote another way by thinking how you can spend money on an exercise program to improve the quality of your life.

> **"The highest use of capital is not to make more money, but to make money do more for the betterment of life."**
> **~Henry Ford**

Take a few minutes today and see where you can save a few dollars that can be spent towards a life-changing exercise program.

CHAPTER 11

Persevere and Become Successful

"I am not judged by the number of times I fail, but by the number of times I succeed; and the number of times I succeed is in direct proportion to the number of times I can fail and keep on trying."

~Tom Hopkins

Perseverance...holding to a course of action or purpose without giving up. Sounds rather simple, doesn't it? But as you probably already know it isn't as easy as it sounds.

According to the health club industry the first 90 days of membership are the most critical when looking toward long-term success with exercise. Most people will drop out during this time period. By the end of the first year of membership, statistics show that 50% of people will quit exercising. To make matters worse I'll bet that percentage is higher for people who exercise at home. Not too promising, is it?

The good news is that you don't have to be one of those statistics. You can be the exception.

I hope that as you read through the chapters of this book you've learned ways to overcome some of the barriers that may have been stalling your efforts to begin or be consistent with an exercise program. But now we come to the barrier that can be the most difficult to overcome. That is the barrier of staying consistent. Persevering through the difficult times. All the other chapters in this book are meaningless unless you can learn to persevere.

Unlock the Power of Perseverance

What will ultimately determine your success with exercise is your ability to persevere. Conrad Hilton once said, "Success seems to be connected with action. Successful people keep moving. They will make mistakes, but they don't quit." This couldn't be closer to the truth when speaking of exercise. You have to keep moving and not give up.

There is no doubt in my mind there will be times when progress comes to a halt. Or a situation comes up in your life resulting in an abandonment of your exercise program for a period of time. There is also the chance of getting injured or sick, making exercise almost impossible for a while.

> **"Success seems to be connected with action. Successful people keep moving. They will make mistakes, but they don't quit."**
> **~Conrad Hilton**

Although many of us want to believe that we are immune to these occurrences, that's not reality. You have to expect and plan for them. The only way to overcome these unexpected occurrences is to persevere through them.

I can't begin to tell you how important it is to persevere. This is what separates success from failure. Without perseverance you will have a very difficult time accomplishing your goals.

With that said, let's take a look at four ideas to help you persevere and be successful with making exercise a part of your life.

1. Know why you are exercising

In order for something to work you need to know why you are doing it. Having a purpose is the fuel that powers perseverance.

In Chapter 7 I wrote about the importance of having a vision to direct you. Having a strong vision gives you that sense of purpose to keep you going when the going gets tough. Then from this vision you establish little goals that get you closer to realizing your vision.

Once you've established your vision or your purpose for starting an exercise program, you need to surround yourself with people who have a strong sense of purpose in their lives as well. They become your strength when you are weak. If you know somebody who has a similar vision and is committed to exercise, then you need to spend time with them. Follow their example.

Finding people to hold you accountable for your exercise program and the goals you've set will greatly contribute to your success.

2. Excuses, excuses...get rid of them!

If I only had a penny for every excuse I've heard over the years I'd have a million dollars. Making excuses can result in a permanent detour on the road to making exercise a part of your life.

When it comes to exercise we make excuses for several reasons. They can come from not knowing what to do, where to carry out the exercise program, how to get started or who will help you. Am I going to stick with it? Can I get my money's worth? Really, what it all boils down to is fear. The fear of uncertainty.

Having fear about this whole exercise thing is understandable. Everybody has a fear of something. Unfortunately these fears, if allowed to dominate your thinking, will stop you before you even get started. You can't let this happen. Eighty percent of the fears we have either never come to pass or are completely out of our control. Yet we focus so much energy on them.

> **Eighty percent of the fears we have either never come to pass or are completely out of our control.**

When it comes to fear there are three ways to handle it. The first way is to completely avoid whatever is causing the fear. In our context, avoiding exercise for fear of not knowing what to do means you don't exercise. What good is that going to be?

You also have the option of hoping the fear will go away over time. This isn't a smart choice either because you may be waiting forever. The longer you wait the more out of shape you become. Waiting isn't the answer.

The only option you have is to stand up to your fear. Take advice from our 32nd President Franklin Delano Roosevelt, when he said, "We have nothing to fear but fear itself." It may not be as difficult as you think. If you are not sure where to start your exercise program, refer to Chapter 3.

Excuses are like armpits...they all stink! There are plenty of willing people, books, and magazines out there to help you face your fears and get started. Making excuses not to exercise boils down to fearing the uncertain. Don't wait for the fear to

> **"You don't face your fears, you stand up to them."**
> **~Unknown author**

go away. Do something about it. George Washington Carver stated, "Ninety-nine percent of failures will come from people who have a habit of making excuses." Be part of the one percent who succeeds!

3. Seek ways to see progress

One of the most powerful motivators for perseverance is seeing progress on a regular basis. Bar none, this is an incredibly important point to consider if you want to persevere and make exercise a part of your life.

When you are able to see small successes on a regular basis it really drives you to keep going. Many people set goals like losing 25 lbs. or being able to bench press 350 lbs. in a specific amount of time. Usually the time period they set is very short. For many people it's a big obstacle to tackle. For some it may seem insurmountable at first. In many cases interest is lost very quickly because it takes too long for the goal to be accomplished. As a result you give up.

Back in Chapter 7, I discussed how to get motivated with exercise by having a vision and setting goals. This process helps you regularly see progress. Here is a recap of what I talked about and how it can be valuable in helping you persevere.

Set goals like simply being able to increase the amount of weight you lift while strength training during the course of one or two weeks. Similarly, for cardiovascular training, set a goal to increase the amount of time you spend on the machine by a couple minutes each week. Record your workouts so you visually see the progress being made. Another simple way to see progress is to just be consistent with your exercise program. It may mean that you exercise twice per week for three months straight. Write down each time you exercise in your daily planner or on a calendar at home. This way you see the consistency in your effort.

It's little things like this I guarantee will make all the difference in the world. Heck, who isn't motivated when progress is constantly being seen? Paul J. Meyer, self-improvement guru and author of *Chicken Soup for the Golden Soul*, says, "Plan your progress carefully; hour-by-hour, day-by-day, month-by-month. Organized activity and maintained enthusiasm are the wellsprings of your power."

Progress can also be seen by getting frequent basic fitness assessments. You can get these at your local health club or have a personal trainer do it for you. The assessments can include body fat percentage, circumference measurements, flexibility, muscular strength and endurance, and aerobic capacity (a measure of your stamina). Have these assessments checked every couple of months.

Finally, you can go to your local hospital and get several medical assessments. These may include blood pressure, full lipid panel (total cholesterol, HDL, LDL, and triglycerides), blood sugar, bone density, or a stress test to measure your cardiovascular health. If you have a family history of high blood pressure, heart disease, diabetes or osteoporosis, I would highly recommend you do this. Consult with your physician to find out how often you should get these checked. The results that come from improvements in these tests are probably ones you will not feel and certainly not see. However, without question they are the most important because they address potentially life-threatening medical issues.

> The best way to persevere is to find ways to seek continuous progress.

If you set goals that are too big you will get discouraged while trying to achieve them. Persevering without progress is difficult. The best way to persevere is to find ways to seek continuous progress.

4. Don't let past failures upset you

Failure at some point in your exercise endeavor is inevitable. Trust me on this one; it's bound to happen.

Have you ever started an exercise program and after only a short time given up? The very reason you are reading this book is because it probably happened to you. If this is true, don't worry about it, just get over it.

This goes back to what we were talking about earlier in the chapter. Maybe you failed at exercise in the past and have a fear that by starting over it will happen again. Ask yourself why you think you failed. Was it that you got bored with it and lost motivation? Maybe you felt too intimidated. Possibly it was because you didn't know what to do and as a result saw no progress.

> **"Use the losses and failures of the past as a reason for action, not inaction."**
> ~ Charles J. Givens

Any of these can be reasons for failure. If it's happened to you, don't despair.

In order to persevere and make exercise a lifelong activity you need to put any failures aside and try again. Take the advice from Charles J. Givens when he said, "Use the losses and failures of the past as a reason for action, not inaction." At least this time you are armed with the material from this book to help out. Remember this: you are only a failure when you give up.

"The Golden Boy of Cycling"

Born on September 18th, 1971, Lance Armstrong is one of the most celebrated contributors to the sport of cycling. This national and world cycling champion, two-time Olympian, and as of 2003, five-time winner of the Tour de France hasn't gone through life without his share of failure and hardships.

Lance began his illustrious career at a young age competing in triathlons. At the age of 13 he won the Iron Kids' Triathlon and by age 16 was a professional triathlete. It didn't take long, however, before Lance found his true love...cycling.

By age 18 he qualified for the junior world championships in Moscow and by age 20 was crowned the U.S. National Amateur Cycling Champion. One year later he had the honor to represent the United States in the 1992 Olympics in Barcelona.

Following the Olympics, Armstrong began competing as a professional. His first race was the 1992 Classico San Sebastian. Although Lance had experienced nothing but success to this point in his career, things changed in a hurry. His first professional race proved to be something he would rather forget. Armstrong finished in last place, 27 minutes behind the leader. Despite the poor performance and with some encouragement from his mother, he didn't quit.

Armstrong's strength and tenacity was evident when the following season rolled around. He won 10 titles including the US PRO Championship, a first-stage victory in the Tour de France, and became the youngest road racing world champion ever.

Over the next two years Armstrong continued his winning ways, chalking up wins in the 1993 Thrift Triple Crown, 1995 Tour Du Pont, and scored a dramatic stage 18 win at the 1995 Tour de France and a victory at the Classico San Sebastian—the same race he finished last at in his first outing as a professional. In 1995 he was named the Velo News American Male Cyclist of the Year.

In 1996, and ranked the number one cyclist in the world, Armstrong's life changed forever. He was diagnosed with advanced testicular cancer that spread to his lungs and brain. He was given less than a 50% chance for recovery. After two surgeries to remove the malignant cancer, an aggressive form of chemotherapy and enormous support from family and friends, Armstrong was on the road to recovery. In fact, just five months after his diagnosis he was back on his bike, training.

Because there was no way I could put this in my own words, the next section of this story is taken directly from the Lance Armstrong Official Website:

Getting cancer was "...the best thing that ever happened to me," Lance said, in relation to the maturity and life focus the disease forced him to face. Throughout this life-threatening ordeal, Lance knew his priorities were changing. His physical well-being, something that had never been challenged, was suddenly fragile. He was given the chance to fully appreciate the blessings of good health, a loving family, and close friends. Lance described his bout with cancer as "a special wake-up call."

In May 1998, just two years after his diagnosis, Armstrong officially returned to the cycling circuit. After a bit of a rough start, he, again, didn't give up and went on to win numerous races that year.

It was in 1999 that he reached the pinnacle of his career by winning the Tour de France for the first time. But as you know it didn't end there. Armstrong's determination and will earned him four more Tour de France victories in as many years, an amazing feat only accomplished by four other riders in history.

Lance Armstrong is a stellar example of someone who could have very easily given up, but didn't. He persevered and as a result experienced great success.

Why Make Exercise
a Part of Your Life?

If I were to ask how you would define success, what would you say? Is it having wealth? Social status? Good health? Certain accomplishments? Moving up the corporate ladder? A great family life? Maybe it is a combination of these things. If I were to ask ten people this question I would probably get ten different answers.

Who doesn't want to be successful? There are hundreds if not thousands of self-help books that teach people how to be successful. There are books on financial success, parenting success, marketing success and even exercise success. Why? Because everybody wants to be successful at what they do.

You purchased this book because you wanted to be successful with exercise. I hope that by reading it you have found ways to overcome the barriers that prevented you from making exercise a part of your life. When you succeed at this you will see changes in your life you never thought possible.

I want you to think of a time when you had the flu or a terrible cold. How did you feel? Horrible, I'm sure. How ambitious did you feel to do anything? The only thing you wanted to do was lie on the couch, right? Feeling unhealthy will cause you to lose your ambition.

I use having the flu as an example of how unmotivated we can be when we're sick. But what if it is more than just the flu? Say you have a chronic disease that causes you to feel under-the-weather all the time. Your condition would greatly influence your potential for success.

Now I'm not saying that just because you exercise that you will never get sick or develop a chronic disease. Anything can happen. However, the likelihood of something happening is far less. Getting involved with exercise and making it a part of your life will help you become more successful.

Try Thinking of Success This Way

One of my all-time favorite authors is John Maxwell. He writes a lot of books on leadership, but one book I thought to be an absolute masterpiece was a book he wrote titled *The Success Journey.*

That book changed my whole thinking on how success is defined. John defines success as a process and not an outcome. You've probably heard the cliché "success is a journey not a destination." He describes success as knowing your purpose in life, growing to meet your potential and sowing the seeds to benefit others.

> "Success is a continuing thing. It is growth and development. It is achieving one thing and using that as a stepping stone to achieve something else."
> ~John Maxwell

The beauty of this definition is that every day you can experience success in your life. Once you know your purpose there is always the opportunity for you to grow. In Maxwell's words, "Success is a continuing thing. It is growth and development. It is achieving one thing and using that as a stepping stone to achieve something else."

You can achieve growth in your profession, family life, and personal life. As you grow in your own life you can help meet the needs of others. There is no final destination defining success. It is a lifetime journey.

Exercise Success Requires a Similar Journey

When you look at the process for describing success in your life it has many similarities to the way you should approach exercise. Like success, exercise should be viewed as a journey. We go through ups and downs, but it is through these things that we become stronger and better equipped to persevere.

With each exercise session you are growing to reach your physical potential. Your daily progress and accomplishments create a feeling of success which breeds growth. This growth carries with it many accomplishments along with many failures, all of which can be used to help others who have struggled in the same way.

The part of exercise that most people overlook is the impact it can have on your entire life. As you move along in your exercise journey, you develop discipline, form habits and create change in your life that will have a positive impact on your family, friends and personal life.

The Decision Is Up to You

It's my hope you learned that exercise isn't a short-term fix. It's not something you do just to look good in your wedding dress, get ready for a class reunion or the summer season. It's a lifetime endeavor. A journey. I encourage you to reread the chapters that discuss the barriers you find most difficult to overcome. Approach each one with a positive attitude. Remember, your attitude determines your altitude.

I want to leave you with a story that is very near and dear to me. It's a story about my son Noah.

Noah entered this world with a bang. After 29 hours of labor my wife had an emergency C-section because Noah decided to wrap the umbilical cord around his neck. Upon delivery we had a surprise...Noah wasn't breathing. After eight minutes of CPR he was revived. Within one hour he stopped breathing for a second time. After being revived the second time he was flown by helicopter to a larger hospital where he would be diagnosed.

It turned out he was born with tracheal esophageal fistula. This meant that his esophagus (food tube) was not attached to his stomach but rather to his trachea (wind pipe). He couldn't eat anything by mouth or it would be aspirated.

The condition required immediate surgery to reattach the esophagus to the stomach in order for him to eat. So 24 hours after his birth he underwent major surgery. The surgery went well; however, several complications required him to spend five weeks in the neonatal intensive care unit before he could come home.

Finally after eight surgeries, 16 months on a feeding tube and many follow-up trips to the hospital, Noah was given a clean bill of health. Noah is now approaching his third birthday and we still occasionally deal with some very minor repercussions; however he is healthy and as active as any other child his age.

We give thanks to the Lord for allowing us to keep Noah and enjoy his playfulness and, sometimes, his sassiness. What an amazing gift we were given.

Through this experience I was able to see the lives of many kids at the Children's Hospital of Milwaukee. Sadly, many of them will never learn to walk, talk, play, or function in a social environment like many of us can. The very things we take for granted are things some can only hope for.

Many of these kids didn't have a choice in life. They were born with a serious condition. They can't choose to do things a little differently in order to change their situation. They will live with it for the remainder of their lives.

My son Noah didn't have a choice whether or not to go through what he did. Thankfully the Lord had a purpose in mind for his life as he does for all of us.

Most of you, on the other hand, do have a choice. You can choose whether or not to enjoy the life you've been given by caring for your body. You have the choice to start an exercise program that can positively impact your life. You have the choice to pursue habits that improve your health.

Or, you can choose to do nothing. To engage in activities that are detrimental to your health. The ball is in your court. What will your decision be?

References

Chapter 1

1. Facts in this chapter are based on information from publications prepared by agencies and offices of the Department of Health an Human Services: the Centers for Disease Control and Prevention; the National Center for Health Statistics; the Office of the Surgeon General of the United States (Physical Activity and Health, 1996; Call to Action to Prevent and Decrease Overweight and Obesity, 2001), and the Office of Disease Prevention and Health Promotion (Healthy People 2010, 2001).

2. Physical Activity Among Adults: United States, 2000. Advance Data No. 333. 23pp. (PIIS) 2003-1250. May 14, 2003.

3. International Health, Racquet & Sportsclub Associaition (IHRSA) Trend Report, April 2003. Volume 10, Number 2.

4. National Research Council, Diet and Health: implications for reducing chronic disease risk. Washington, D.C.; National Academy Press, 1989.

5. Patrick Amend, Countdown to Get Active America, *Club Business International*, February 2004. pp. 60-64.

6. Cancer Statistics 2004. A Presentation from the American Cancer Society 2004.

7. Jennifer Warner, Obesity Costs Rival Smoking. May 15, 2003. www.my.webmd.com

Chapter 2

1. Steve Young, *Great Failures of the Extremely Successful* (Los Angeles: Tallfellow Press, 2002).

2. Walt Disney: Long Biography, www.justdisney.com

3. Time 100: The Wright Brothers, www.time.com

4. Carol Krucoff, Why You're Not Exericsing, www.familyfun.com

5. Ace and Consumer Reports Magazine Review the Latest Infomercial Products, www.acefitness.org

Chapter 3

1. International Health, Racquet & Sportsclub Association (IHRSA) Trend Report, July 2003. Volume 10, Number 3.

2. International Health, Racquet & Sportsclub Association (IHRSA) Trend Report. October 2003. Volume 10, Number 4.

3. Featured articles, In Search of Personal Training: a look at styles around the world. August 2003, www.fit-pro.com

4. Brian McDermott, Certification: A Connection to Competence. *Fitness Management,* December 2002.

Chapter 4

1. Fast Facts on Osteoporosis, www.nof.org

2. International Health, Racquet & Sportsclub Association (IHRSA) Trend Report, July 2002. Volume 9, Number 3.

Chapter 5

1. Joel Schwarz, How to keep up with those New Year's resolutions, researchers find commitment is the secret to success, www.washington.edu, December 23, 1997.

2. Rick Pitino, *Success is a Choice* (New York: Broadway Books, 1997).

3. Bill Phillips and Michael D'Orso, *Body for Life* (New York: Harper Collins Publisher, 1999), 100-101.

4. Barbara A. Behm, Exercise Success: Willpower is Part of the Picture, *Fitness Management*, October 2002.

5. Ecclesiastes 4:9-10 NIV.

Chapter 6

1. In Broadband Households, the Internet has Nearly Caught Up With TV and Radio in Battle for the Consumer's Time, www.screenwriters.scriptmania.com, September 22, 2000.

2. I-M Lee, Physical Activity and Cancer Prevention—Data from Epidemiologic Studies, *Medicine & Science in Sports & Exericse*, Volume 35 (11), November 2003. pp. 1823-1827.

3. Anxiety, exercise, exercise and stress, exercise and anxiety, www.holisticonline.com

4. Patrick M. Morely, *The Seven Seasons of a Man's Life* (Grand Rapids: Zondervan), pg. 95.

5. Steve Young, *Great Failures of the Extremely Successful* (Los Angeles: Tallfellow Press, 2002), pp. 41-44.

6. John Maxwell, *Leadership 101* (Nashville: Thomas Nelson Publishers, 2002), pg. 49.

7. Stephen R. Covey, *The Seven Habits of Highly Effective People* (New York: Simon & Schuster, 1989), pg. 151.

8. Vince Lombardi, Jr. and John Q. Baucom, *Baby Steps to Success* (Lancaster: Starburst Publishing, 1997).

9. Krs Edstrom, *Healthy, Wealthy & Wise* (Los Angeles: Soft Stone Publishing, 1999).

10. Fitness Industry Statistics, www.sportsspin.com

Chapter 7

1. Zig Ziglar, *Over the Top* (Nashville: Thomas Nelson Publishers, 1994), pp. 110-111.

2. Charles Stuart Platkin, Find that one exercise you enjoy; focus on fun, www.honoluluadvertiser.com, October 29, 2003.

3. Seven Habits of Highly Fit People—Exercise at Bellaonline, www.bellaonline.com

4. Rick Pitino, *Success is a Choice* (New York: Broadway Books, 1997).

5. Vince Lombardi, Jr. and John Q. Baucom, *Baby Steps to Success* (Lancaster: Starburst Publishing, 1997), pg. 62.

6. Stephen R. Covey, *First Things First* (New York: Simon & Schuster, 1994).

Chapter 8

1. International Health, Racquet & Sportsclub Association (IHRSA) Trend Report. October 2003. Volume 10, Number 4.

2. Sameh Fahmy, Curve appeal, www.tennessean.com, February 17, 2004.

3. John Maxwell, *Becoming a Person of Influence* (Nashville: Thomas Nelson Publishers, 1997), pg. 49.

4. Brian Tracey, <u>Cultivating Your Self-Esteem</u>, www.emotional-success.com

5. Dr. Phil McGraw, *The Ultimate Weight Solution* (New York: The Free Press, 2003), pp. 66-67.

Chapter 9

1. www.healthstatus.com

2. <u>Chores that add up</u>, www.ajc.com, Atlanta Journal Constitution.

3. International Health, Racquet & Sportsclub Association (IHRSA) Trend Report, July 2002. Volume 9, Number 3.

4. <u>Overcome Exercise Plateaus & Boredom with Cross Training</u>, www.prima-fit.com

Chapter 10

1. Dave Ramsey, *The Total Money Makeover* (Nashville: Thomas Nelson Publishers, 2003).

Chapter 11

1. Lance Armstrong—A Biography, www.lancearmstrong.com

0-595-32260-3

www.ingramcontent.com/pod-product-compliance
Lightning Source LLC
Chambersburg PA
CBHW061257280526
45784CB00002B/792